The Fluid Dynamics of Craniosacral Therapy: Foundational Biodynamics

By Dominique Clothiaux

The Fluid Dynamics of Craniosacral Therapy : Fundamental Biodynamics

Published 2024 by Birth & Biodynamics
Charlottesville, Virginia
© 2024 Dominique Clothiaux

ISBN: 9798873476909
Also available as an e-book

This book offers general information for interest only and does not constitute or replace individualized professional craniosacral therapy or medical care and advise. Whilst every effort has been made to ensure the accuracy and currency of the information presented, herein the author accepts no liability or responsibility for any loss or damage caused, or thought to be caused, by decisions made based upon the information stated in this book and recommends that you use it in conjunction with other trusted sources of information

The Fluid Dynamics of Craniosacral Therapy: Foundational Biodynamics

Table of Contents

Chapter 1: History of Craniosacral Therapy: The History of Osteopathic Medicine Equals the Beginning of Craniosacral Therapy ....page 7

Chapter 2: Evolution ....page 19

Chapter 3 Fundamental Principles behind Primary Respiration ....page 26

Chapter4: Subtle Body and Soul ....page 42

Chapter 5 The Orientation of the Embryo ....page 53

Chapter 6 : Fascial Dynamics: How One Part Affects the Whole ....page 72

Chapter 7: Anatomy of the Autonomic Nervous System ....page 77

Chapter 8: The Source Behind Craniosacral Therapy ....page 91

Chapter 9: Anatomical and Physiological Realms: The Nervous System Tissue and its Relationships to the Primary Respiratory Mechanism ....page 98

Chapter 10: Cranial Nerves ....page 117

Chapter 11: How to Work with Still Points ....page 163

Chapter 12: The Physics of Health ....page 173

About the Author......................................page 186

In honor of the journey that lead me down the path of understanding imprints and the miraculous ability to heal my life to resilience.

Dedicated to my Grandfather Clothiaux who instilled a love and belief for the mystery beyond what can be seen nor completely understood.

Chapter One

History of Craniosacral Therapy

The History of Osteopathic Medicine Equals the Beginning of Craniosacral Therapy

Dr Andrew Taylor Stills

Craniosacral Therapy first emerged out of the beginnings of Osteopathic Medicine between 1864 and the 1930s. The founder of Osteopathic Medicine was Dr. Andrew Taylor Stills who resided in the southeast region of the United States. Born in Virginia, he lived most of his young adulthood in Kansas where his family founded Baker University. Later he moved on to found the American School of Osteopathy (now called A.T. Stills University) of Kirksville, Missouri in 1892. The son of a Methodist minister and physician, Stills spent

Dr. Andrew Taylor Stills' Journey:

- He set out to study the mechanism behind our tissues.
- He discovered that all systems of the body are connected.
- Any dysfunction in either system would affect the other.
- Viscera (organs) are connected to soma (connective tissue, joints, nerves, blood, lymphatic vessels and basically all tissues and fluid).
- He discovered that by palpating the body in a quite slowed down manner he could actually trace how tissue was affecting other tissue.
- He also came to understand that there was a kind of life force which organized the body that was beyond what could be seen, measured or completely understood. He named this life force 'The Breath of Life'.

Other contributions:
- He was the first to identify the human immune system and developed techniques to stimulate it naturally.
- He was the first to welcome women and minorities into medical schools.
- He predicted that the United States would have a major drug addiction problem by the end of the 19th century of physicians did not stop over prescribing addictive medications.
- He believed doctors should study prevention as well as cures.

much of his youth traveling and assisting his father on home visits. He became a military surgeon during the civil war.

His ideas about the healing process came through great trauma. After losing two wives (one to child birth complications and the other to pneumonia) then watching three of his children die of spinal meningitis in 1864, he began to doubt the methods of allopathic medicine. He questioned whether the human capacity to heal was locked inside the body rather than something that could be treated by medication. He asked his heart, "In sickness has God left man in the world of guessing?" Having been a lifelong observer and lover of nature, he decided "God is not a guessing God, but a God of truth. All his works, spiritual and material, are harmonious. His law of life is absolute. So wise a God places the remedy within the material house in which the spirit dwells." Inspired by this truth, he set out to study the mechanisms behind our physiology which became the ongoing study and foundation behind true Osteopathic philosophy which would be carried on by those truly interested in the living organism.

He began by going back to study human anatomy and spent much time with the bones. Dr Stills discovered that through the connective tissue layers in the body, all things were connected. Viscera (organs) are connected to all levels of soma (connective tissue, joints, nerves, blood, lymphatic vessels and basically all tissues and fluids of the body as a whole). Any dysfunction in

either system would affect the other. Furthermore, he discovered that by palpating the body he could actually trace how the tissue was affected the whole through his keen sense and understanding of the living body. He also came to understand whole heartedly that there was a kind of life force which organized the body that was beyond what could be seen, measured or even completely understood. He named this life force 'The Breath of Life.

Dr William G. Sutherland

Dr Stills work was continued by one of his students, Dr. William G. Sutherland, who discovered that there was a subtle, palpable oscillation, which the Breath of Life engenders, called the 'Primary Respiratory Mechanism'. This discovery of Primary Respiration and its mechanism ended up being the most outstanding contribution in the history of physiology. This subtle motion, which is found most predominately in the tissues of the central nervous system but also exists throughout the entire body, is what organizes all tissue and function in the body. He first identified the manifestation of these movements in the cranial bones, theorizing that the sutures must not fuse together completely and that somehow the movement of the bones had something to do with vitality and health. He experimented with his own skull by designing a leather helmet that would put pressure on individual cranial bones and which he wore for extended periods of time. He documented the effect of these self experiments and documented a significant difference in his health and state of well being. Through these experiments he experienced various states of chronic depression, hysteria, headaches, sinus imbalances and digestive disorders to name a few. He then began to palpate his patients skull in order to help him diagnose and to investigate even further if gentle manipulation could ease ailments. He had much success practicing medicine in this way. His speculation was that this movement of primary respiration, which had nothing to do with the respiratory breath or the heart beat, was part of the physical manifestation of the breath of life and essential to life itself. In fact, somewhere along his studies and experiments he resuscitated a drowning victim simply by pumping the temporal bones like the gills of a fish. His instinct to move the temporal bones in that manner came from studying the squamous suture which surrounds the temporals. To him the bones literally looked like the gills of a fish and his theory was that it was because they actually moved like the gills of a fish. The pumping action of the temporal bones he was able to achieve during the resuscitation kept the primary respiratory mechanism moving through the fluid circulation in and around the brain. This solidified all the work in his studies indicated that the movements of the breath of life and the movement of the cranial bones where one. Towards the end of his life, Dr Sutherland lived by the ocean and came to believe that these subtle motions in the body actually had many layers to their movement similar to the tides of the ocean.

Dr. William G. Sutherland's Journey:

- Discovered the 'Primary Respiratory Mechanism' - a subtle, palpable oscillation found in all fluid tissues of the body which the Breath of Life engenders. This movement was first recognized in the cerebral spinal fluid around the brain; however, it is present in ALL fluid throughout the body and has been scientifically noted in all cellular fluid called cellular oscillation. This discovery is the single most outstanding discovery in the history of physiology.

- Named the different layers of movement present in Primary Respiration as the Tides.

Essentially, the history behind Osteopathic Medicine represents the beginning of craniosacral work. The whole foundation which Osteopathic Doctors originally based their practice and understanding of medicine came from "listening" to a person's system. They did this by placing their hands on the patient to feel how one part or system was affecting the other systems. They used their palpation skills as a diagnostic tool AND a mode of treatment. It used to be that when you visited your local Osteopathic Doctor (DO), he/she would listen to the patients' health complaints then place their hands on the patient to literally feel into the different tissues layers and be able to trace how the entire body was integrating the whole experience. They would then diagnosis and treat from what they were able to perceive through their hands. The ordering of labs, screening and tests were just to confirm what they were sensing. They always relied on the movement they noticed in the living cells by listening to 'The Breath of Life' first and letting that be a guiding force in all treatments.

Unfortunately, in today's world there are few Osteopaths that place their hands on a patient as a part of treatment protocol. As we have entered the new millennium, there has been a slow death of true Osteopathy in the United States. Medical doctors and osteopathic doctors are virtually indistinguishable from one another. Though, osteopathic doctors do get a formal training in manual techniques and are encouraged to be mindful of the body as an integrative whole comprised of body, mind and spirit. They became disguised within the medical field as ordinary medical doctors.

The mainstream direction of the osteopathic education route in the United States is no longer interested in the living physiology. The general movement of the American Medical Associations have became about politics and interest in profit. Part of the recovery process coming out of the great depression focused on enterprise and building a strong economy of systematic money making. The rise of allopathic medicine which emerged around the same time as osteopathic medicine became the primary western medical model of care. Its focus is primarily treating with medication and relies on intervention from an outside force to create the healing process. Through the birth of allopathic medicine came the pharmaceutical industry that quickly built up with the help of the United States government which in turn began orchestrating the direction of modern medicine offering funds towards scientific research that were the interest of the industrial machine. This system of industry and government in terms of health care is still strongly in place and it now includes an even more politically complicated arena of money making business. In trust health care in our country has become less about facilitating the healing process and more about a consumer industry. There is very little money to be made if patients can heal from the inside out, using their own internal resources.

The general mind set of our civilization has chosen to focus on what can only be measured through what is physically seen. This attitude spread beyond medicine and has integrated through the shaping of the industrial age and how consumerism has maintained its dominance through the later part of history. Few corners of our western medical society are truly interested in continuing research into that which is alive. The same can be said for society as a whole. Environmental issues are screaming at us but the modern comforts and consumerism is still the driving force. To walk in respect of nature and the natural process in our world require a kind of sacred stillness and patience that would take away from all the big money making machines of our times.

Philosophically, most of the models taught in anatomy and physiology courses are based on information coming out of the study of cadavers anyways and are Cartesian in nature. Cartesianism is the name given to the philosophical and scientific system that only verifies what can be seen with the naked eye. Cadavers are dead dried tissue and nothing like the living body. To study the living physiology and to understand the mystery that lives underneath our tissues is very difficult to inquire within a controlled environment such as a lab. The breath of life is extremely intelligent. It always knows when it is being watch and it will act accordingly.

The study of physiology and the living mechanism behind our bodies entails quieting and slowing down while observing the living world and being present with another person. There have been actual scientific studies into the living movement of the tissues. Tufts University biologists in August 2012 recorded for the first time in history a bioelectric signal that is physiologically necessary for normal formation of the embryo. Capturing this movement of the living physiology on film was an impressive feat because the Breath of Life always knows when it is being watched and will act accordingly. The master intelligence behind our physiology makes experiments difficult and requires a kind of patience and openness that is unlikely to be funded by the types of institutions that could properly prove how this living mechanism can unlock the healing process. Institutions that could potentially prove funding would only be interested in how they could use the research to manipulate through the development of medicines or other means that could add to the stock of their system. To clarify more simply, there is much about how our bodies and the living world that is beyond what could be seen, measured or completely understood. It would seem there is a master intelligence behind it all. To try and harness what is so brilliant would be like trying to master God when all it needs is to be nurtured with divine presence and acknowledgement in order for the magic of our physiology to speak what is there then to begin its shifting process back towards the health.

Furthermore, there was a division between Osteopathic Medicine and Osteopathy in the 1960s. The American Osteopathic Association wanted to separate the medical aspects of osteopathic medicine with the hands on portion of the work. Liability reasons have been the main rationalization behind why the field of medicine wanted to move away from interacting with patients through touch, even though touch and the relational field are essential for the recovery and healing process. Humans are biologically wired for connection! Osteopaths are non-physicians and focus primarily of the hands-on techniques that was birthed out of Osteopathic medicine. Today, European Osteopaths are instructed in osteopathic manipulation (or manual therapy) and are not trained in surgery, pharmacology and the like. They are non-physicians and more like manual therapist. Osteopaths are not permitted to practice under licensure in the United States but rather can physical therapist, massage therapist or chiropractic can practice certain osteopathic techniques under their licensure. Licensed osteopathic doctors may also practice osteopathy. However, few American osteopathic medical schools teach in-depth hands-on modalities. If they do they are elective courses and many osteopathic doctors are not taught the art of using the hands as a primary diagnostic tool unless they seek out special training. Hence, the death of "true" Osteopathic Medicine.

Because Craniosacral Therapy is so experiential and unique for each patient, this disinterest from its originators actually makes it more accessible to be truly studied and understood in a non-systemized way through alternative medicine. Thus, allowing the creativity of the health we carry within our bodies to express itself with tremendous freedom within and without. In essence, we must allow the practice of listening to be the ultimate teacher in the healing process and in field of Biodynamic Craniosacral Therapy we can do just that. The legacy of craniosacral therapy that has been left to the world, by genuine osteopaths, may be the greatest gift to the medical field. Those who have held on to the original integrity of osteopathic medicine are indeed birthing even greater understandings. Since its humble beginning, it has been a continual journey into how to work with the living physiology and how to unlock a person's own natural healing process in the face of disease, trauma, illness and chronic pain.

~

Other Osteopaths who Continued Research into Craniosacral Therapy

Dr. Rollin Becker, DO – was a student of William Sutherland. He emphasized the importance of treatment being guided by a 'listening' approach and the value in recognizing and harnessing the potential of self-corrective mechanisms within the body, using terms such as 'physician within' and 'silent partner' to convey this simple, but highly practical and important philosophical concept.

Dr. Viola Frymann, DO – founded the Osteopathic Center for Children. She taught craniosacral to dentists and advocated craniosacral treatment for neurological development problems.

Dr. John Upledger, DO – founded the Upledger Institute in the 1970s. He was the first to bring craniosacral work outside osteopathic medicine and has been critical in the creation of a defined <u>craniosacral therapy profession</u> that practices outside of the osteopathic framework. He confirmed that the bones of the cranium do move through intense research and experiments.

Dr. James Jealous, DO – developer, researcher and refiner of Biodynamic Cranial Osteopathy, professor of the New England College of Osteopathic Medicine and the main osteopath who continues to explore and research the legacy of A.T. Stills and William Sutherland.

Franklyn Sills – is not an osteopathic doctor but a cranial osteopath and contemplative psychologist who bridges Biodynamic Cranial Osteopathy and Contemplative or Buddhist Psychology for those outside of Osteopathic Medicine. He is the founder of the Biodynamic Craniosacral Association, a world-wide organization, which offers the highest known credentialing program available in Craniosacral Therapy outside of Osteopathic Craniosacral Therapy.

There are 4 schools of thought on Craniosacral Therapy

Biomechanical or Functional CranioSacral Therapy – This follows Upledgers' work and consists of following the same protocols for each patient, working more with the dysfunction/ imbalance or inertia present in the tissue. This type of therapy works to mechanically fix the imbalance through regulating the Cranio Rhythmic Impulse (CRI). It is based on the idea that when things are aligned things function better. It focuses on aligning the system in an anatomical way.

Visionary Craniosacral Therapy – This is shamanic type of craniosacral therapy that works more with energetic qualities of the patient. Milne Hughes is the main developer of this work.

Biodynamic Craniosacral Therapy is the extension of Osteopathic research and understanding of the craniosacral system. It works to extenuate the Health in the physiology in the body by listening to the various tides of the Breath of Life in the whole system. It is a technique that focuses on ways to support the Health that is already there and trusting the Breath of Life and the Tides to do all the work of healing.

Biodynamic Cranial Osteopathy is only available to those who have trained as Osteopathic doctors and encompasses biomechanical, functional and biodynamic craniosacral therapy.

~

The field of Biodynamic Craniosacral Therapy and Biodynamic Cranial Osteopathy is essentially the continuation of Dr A.T. Stills research. It is the part of Osteopathic Medicine that has tried to completely cohere and evolve its understanding of living physiology in terms of how to effectively treat imbalance by assisting the body's own natural healing mechanisms to make changes toward health. Only through the art of deep listening always careful not to disturb, these practices have continued with great dedication to the stillness and the mystery.

Chapter Two

Evolution

The underlying principle behind craniosacral therapy is that there is a "healing intelligence" within the body that maintains health at all times. Health is always there. It is an ever present force in our Being. It is neither born nor does it die. It is constant. In our soma, health is forever organizing around the original embryological "blue print" of our making which anatomically begins with conception. How health organizes in our bodies is modified from the original intention of that embryological Blue Print, by our life experiences and by our genetics. All parts affect the whole this is the concept behind the osteopathic term "inherent health".

Biodynamic craniosacral therapy facilitates the body's own natural healing processes in restoring health and balance. It is a gentle, non-invasive method of treatment that has proven to be effective in treating a wide range of medical problems associated with pain, trauma, illness and dysfunction. It is a subtle yet profound approach to healing.

A biodynamic craniosacral therapist works to support the health that is already there, not necessarily the place where trauma occurs or where is lay manifest in the physical body. The wider known 'Biomechanical CranioSacral' therapy is centered more around structural balance and integrity while also finding a way to align the body through 'craniosacral manipulations'. A biodynamic craniosacral therapist has a deep knowledge of manual therapy, but actually works to hold the entire aspect of inherent health in their awareness and works to make health and the underling Intelligence stronger in the body. This is done by helping the cellular tissues to settle and trusting the breath of life and the physiological tides. Biodynamic craniosacral therapy is centered on helping the physiology to find Stillness where it can recharge and gain access to its original state. By doing so the body can release holding patterns associated with trauma, illness and other chronic conditions. If unwinding happens in a session, the therapist works to slow things down and to 'resource' the trauma through dynamic stillness. Therapist knowledge of how to work with the primary respiratory mechanism comes from a deep understanding of anatomy, fluid dynamics, embryology, and Buddhist psychology. The therapist listens to the entire system with his/her hands along with their entire being through a mindfulness based practice of presence. This deep listening combined with facilitation of dynamic stillness is what helps the body to remember the health and intelligence that is already there.

What happens in a Biodynamic Craniosacral session? The client will usually come in presenting with their condition or complaint in the foreground, or in the center of their consciousness, with the blue print or underlying health out of reach from their internal resources. The therapist provides a neutral and non-intrusive field that will reflect and perceive wholeness in the client's system. Within the therapist's neutral field they will include in their awareness the whole person that contains the story, the condition, the history in the system as well as the anatomy and physiology, the health, the blueprint and the mid-line point of balance in the tissues. After some time, the client's physiology will begin to remember space, option, health, blueprint and wholeness all the while beginning to present signs of resource. Resource is important in the healing process because that is where the body can change its state through a process called transmutation. Transmutation is where form is organized, fluid cohesion and integration can happen through the building of potency on the cellular tissue. This potency brings movement to the physical tissue from a place called "Dynamic Stillness". When these elements occur (accurate reflection, midline awareness, resource, dynamic stillness and potency), the body can experience healing sustained on a permanent level, because it has moved on its own, in its own time with the support of the therapist.

Craniosacral Therapy is not energy work rather it is based on the physical body and its subtle expressions of movement. In order for the practitioner to feel these movements and to perceive the whole system of expression he/she must sit quietly "listening" with a quiet mind and hands that are "thinking, feeling, seeing and knowing". The fluids of the body are very intelligent and it is only when the client is in a relaxed state, feeling safe and secure and supported that the motilities of the body can show the practitioner their true nature.

What they listen for is the embryology patterns, the nervous system functions, the organ motility, bone and 'fascial tensile fields' all of which are driven by the fluid system. Within the fluid system there are very subtle rhythms that have many different layers to them. Those layers are called "Tides" because they move throughout the body just the same as the different tidal layers of the ocean and all bodies of water on Earth. These tides give potential for the potency of breath of life to be carried into every cell, and tissue in the body, bringing life and health to the surface.

Biodynamic craniosacral therapy also works with the relational field in a way that creates a safe therapeutic atmosphere before a client gets on the table. Craniosacral work can transform the process of psychology when treating chronic conditions and

---

Primary Respiratory Mechanism

- Subtle motion

- Found in all the body systems

- Is present in cellular oscillation and is the fundamental quality of fluid dynamics

- Most noticeable in the movement of the cerebral spinal fluid up and down the spine and within the movement of the cranial bones

- Organized around the "Original Blue Print" of the Breath of Life originating during our embryological beginnings and continues to operate throughout life

- Polyrhythmic

---

disease. The movement of the breath of life and primary respiration mechanism alone is what preserves the transformation process of the psychology. Psychotherapeutic dialogue is not

essential to the therapeutic process of the inherent treatment plan and can be more of an interruption to the therapeutic process. However, the degree of safety between the therapist and client is essential to the healing process which is established by the therapist's ability help the client settle into mindful awareness of the body and its sensations. It is also helpful for the therapist to understand and reflect the clients' deepest intention for the work and to help establish resource for the client, using the relational field.

One thing that is so amazing about the effects of Biodynamic Craniosacral Therapy is that it is like the gift that keeps on giving! Often the real change in the physiology will happen weeks after a session. The body will move and adjust itself just at a speed that is right for the individual person. The healing process is a slow process and if the body has a chance to correct itself in its own time, then the changes that occur will stay.

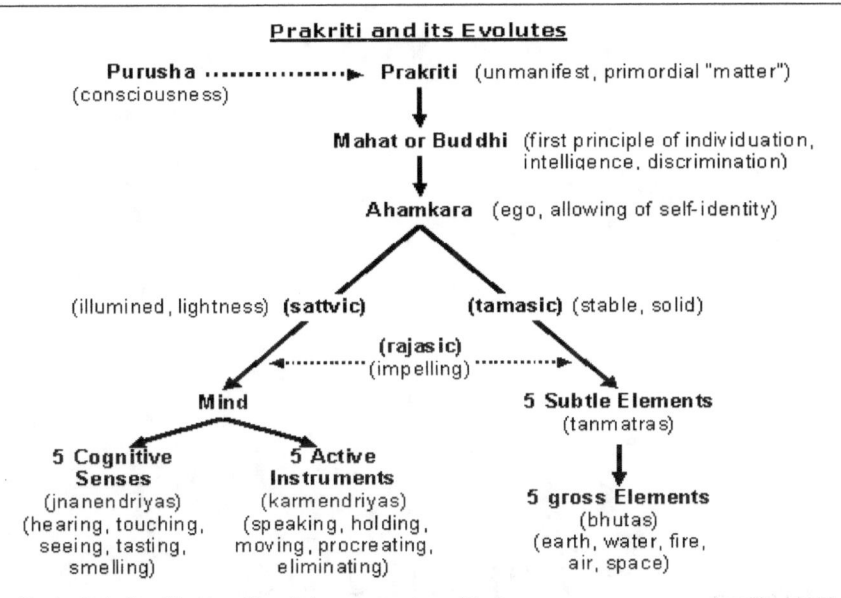

Chart adapted/modified from Yoga Sutras commentary of U. Arya.

Chapter Three

Fundamental Principles behind Primary Respiration

Primary Respiration is the inherent motion present in our physiology. It organizes all the rhythms and fluids of the body. It's a subtle, palpable oscillation and is found most predominantly in the tissues of the central nervous system, although it exists throughout the entire body. This motion is what organizes all of the tissues and functions in the body. Acting as single unit of function, this motion actually arises from the force we call the Breath of Life. The principle movement of this mysterious force has an organizing effect on the fluids that is carried out through the body via primary respiration. Somewhere between where the breath of life emerges and the movement of primary respiration, is the body's natural self-correcting force which heals all injuries and traumas.

Primary Respiration is the most intrinsic motion within our physiology. Its motion is present in cellular oscillation and is the fundamental quality of fluid dynamics. This sacred movement moves in a fluctuating pattern of coming in and going back out like the tides of the ocean, all the while organizing the tissues to create balance between its original intention, its experience with the present moment and the history of all that came before. In essence, primary respiration is the physical manifestation of the biodynamic potency behind the breath of life. It does this by organizing all functions of all the bones and systems in the body (muscular, visceral (organs), nervous system, cardiovascular, etc) all according to both our original essence and life experiences.

Primary Respiration is the organizing force of tissue. But what organizes Primary Respiration? The many layers and the origin of primary respiration are found in the universal laws of fluid dynamics, embryology, the bioelectric field and the movement of the tides.

```
5 Core Aspects of Primary Respiration

    1.  The inherent fluctuation of the cerebrospinal
        fluid (CSF)

    2.  The inherent motility of the central nervous
        system (CNS)

    3.  The motility of the dural sheaths and the
        reciprocal tension membranes (RTM)

    4.  The motion of the cranial bones, the
        involuntary motion of the sacrum between the
        iliac bones on the pelvis

    5.  Motility of the visceral system (organs)
```

Fluid Dynamics

Epigenetic is a biological term that refers to how genes express throughout the life experience and between generations. Genetics are stable during cell division and are not involved in the underlying sequencing of DNA characteristics of the organism during the formation of its conception. Meaning the genes are laid down but they do not become active until later on in life. What is known as the primal health period, the time between conception to through the first year of life, determines which genes get turned on and off later on in life. Hence one of the biggest discovers of the genome project was the identification that life experience and exposure to stress particularly in the primal health period is what determines which genes get activated in a person's DNA.

The laws of fluid dynamics are epigenetic (they never change and are always the same in every situation). The epigenetic law within fluid dynamics and the behavior of water exist within underlying sequencing of its movement and behavior universally throughout the planet. The basic laws of fluid dynamics are found in our embryological beginnings. The fluid dynamic understanding of biodynamic craniosacral therapy is a particular approach in the study of the natural and creative forces that organize the human body. The forces that are found throughout the natural world are the same forces that we carry within our physiology. They include a subtle ordering principle that drives the creation, development and maintenance of all systems. Within the expression of these forces is a polyrhythmic movement that is constant and palpable, moving in cycles known as primary respiration. This movement is omnipresent in all living organisms and it moves in a natural expansion-contraction pattern that is very different than the respiratory breath and the heart beat. Interactions such as therapeutic treatment with the movements present in craniosacral understanding can have remarkable health benefits.

As embryos we are made purely from water dynamics. We begin from water and we are formed from water. Water is the essential element in order for life to exist. It is the perfect medium of which the breath of life can interface. But how does water move to form that which we become?

The dynamics of water are the same in every situation. When two polar opposites meet in water dynamics they do not collide but move together to build a vortex. It is the movement of fluid within fluid encased in the boundaries of a sac that creates the shape of the embryo. The expression of fluidity is the foundation of the embryo. We see in the basic laws of water dynamics that when a container is injected with water it creates a simple form of movement that is exactly similar to part of the movements of our formation into embryos as well as the formation of other forms of living matter such as plants and other nonhuman embryos. The process of "Becoming" is created from water in motion: water and motion create life.

Primitive Streak

The Primitive Streak is the first embryonic axis around which our tissues are formed. It is a bioelectric streak of light that appears around the fourteenth day after conception. It is a mysterious streak of light that has a sparkly quality similar to phosphorescence. Its development establishes bilateral symmetry for the body to form around, creating a fulcrum called the mid-line.

The streak disappears after full development of the embryo, but we carry remnant cells within the vertebral discs of the spine. This subtle mid-line is the original blueprint of our Being and is the axis of travel for the *Craniosacral Tidal Movements* throughout the entirety of life. It is the master organizer of how 'The Breath of Life' interacts with our tissue AND how we incorporate all of our experiences within all systems in the body - nervous system, organ system, muscular system, fluid system, etc.

Primitive Streak

- After conception the sperm and the egg begin cell division.

- The Primitive Streak appears on the 14th day after conception and is a mysterious streak of light with a sparkly quality similar to phosphorescence.

- Its development establishes bilateral symmetry for the body to form around, creating a fulcrum called the energetic mid-line in the adult but it is the site where the Notochord is formed around. The notochord is a rod like cord of cells that forms the chief axial supporting structure of the body during embryonic development.

One of the most distinguishing features of the mechanics of Primary Respiration is its emphasis on the mid-line. Ventral mid-line pertains to the front or anterior of the spinal cord which is along the remnants of the Primitive Streak. It is the major axis of development within the embryo, as well as the major organizing force behind the movement of biodynamic potencies within the adult human being.

In utero, primary respiration expresses as an uprising force where the primitive streak and notochord form. It is the ordering axis for the generation of form in the embryo. Its continues to function in that same way as a natural orientation point for all the tissues of the body to be organized. This mid-line is where the Breath of Life can travel in a way that can organize. The mid-line is anatomically centered through the center of our bodies along the line of the front part of the spine, through the vertebral bodies. The fluid action that of ventral mid-line is sometimes call 'The Fountain Spray of Life' because the movement of the Breath of Life here can be palpated as moving upward from the coccyx, through the vertebral bodies, to the occiput, and spraying out through the sphenoid. In the same way it was formed, it continues to be a major organizing pathway for the Breath of Life to travel to bring balance and organization to the tissues within the body.

Bio-Electric Field

In August 2012, Tufts University biologists have reported that bioelectrical signals are necessary for normal head and facial formation in an all organisms. However, Biodynamic Craniosacral Therapists, have been aware of this information for quite some time.

This bioelectric field is what organizes form all together. As an embryo, we begin our formation in a manner similar to a mineral - by growing out into the world in a somewhat disorganized fashion. Then magically a bioelectric streak of light appears, creating a mid-line and the whole growth pattern of the embryo changes into something more organized. It becomes more organized by initiating the movements of our growing pattern into spirals by pulling in the cells inward and organizing each cell by assigning into its place in the body. The embryo also folds as a result of the energetic field coming through.

The world is alive and we are in relationship with it. Science is just beginning to understand living physiology. All life grows and moves in spirals. Our being is not separate from all cosmic forces at play. We are creatures that are surrounded by an environmental field. We are made mostly of water. Our environment (which is also a part of us both energetically and physically) organizes a fluid body where the energetic qualities of our being and feeling bodies (autonomic nervous system) meet. Our physical body is where the metaphorical and more solid essences manifest into form. All these layers are grounded by a deep and knowing Stillness out of which the potency to drive and organize all these forces at once. When we look at the body this way it becomes clear. Form is organizing the fluid within the field AND form becomes denser as it comes to center of the physical.

The body has many different rhythms and when you bring it together you have biodynamic forces. The expression of them all is a reflection of what is happening in the parasympathetic and sympathetic nervous system. This is in essence what we are listening to and helping to balance during a craniosacral therapy session.

Biodynamic Craniosacral Therapy is a particular approach to the study of the natural and creative forces that organize the human body. The forces that are found throughout the natural world are the same forces that we carry within our physiology. They include a subtle ordering principle that drives the creation, development and maintenance of all systems. Within the expression of these forces is a polyrhythmic movement that is stable and palpable, moving in cycles and spirals known as Primary Respiration. This movement is omnipresent in all living organisms and it moves in a natural expansion-contraction pattern that is very different than the respiratory breath and the heart beat. Interactions with the movements present in craniosacral understanding can have remarkable health benefits.

Water

The human body is composed mostly of water: 75% in a new born which decreases subtly over time to about 50% in old age. The average adult's body is composed of about 67% water.

Water is extremely resonant and will change its molecular structure according to its surrounding environment. Indigenous elders from all over the globe have been telling us for eons to pray with water if we want to change the state of health inside our bodies AND on our planet. In the early 1990's a Japanese scientist Masaru Emoto proved that water changes it molecules to match the energetic vibration of that which surrounds a particular vessel or body of water. He published this discovery in his book 'Message in Water'.

As with water the fluid in our bodies also reacts to the energetic vibrations in our environment, such as speed, stress and trauma by becoming condensed and rigid. Hence, structures in our tissues change in different situations.

Tides

Within Primary Respiration there are different layers of organized movement that ripple through our fluid body. These movements are subtle and are experienced as the Cranial Rhythmic Impulse (CRI), Mid-tide, Long-tide, and Dynamic Stillness. The rhythms are the movements of our physiology and are simultaneously present within us all. The state of the nervous system and how much subtle body awareness we have will indicate what layer we experience these rhythms.

Tidal Movements of the Breath of Life

Tidal movements flow along the mid-line and are the carrier of the intention of The Breath of Life to our tissue. It is best understood if you view the body as large body of water where there are many different layers of movement: the top layer having the most movement that organizes around the outside forces and the bottom layer being still and calm.

Cranial Rhythmic Impulse (CRI) –CRI moves much like the movement of waves on top of a large body of water. Its rate is very fast and choppy and not so much in unison with the whole body. This is the layer of motility where inertia exists; it does not organize around the mid-line and the original blue print. This movement corresponds to the bone and tissue movements of the body while orienting to what is happening in our day to day lives.

Mid-Tide- The rate is about 8 seconds inhalation and 8 seconds exhalation. It moves in unison with the whole in relation to the mid-line of the body. This movement corresponds to fluctuations of fluid and the integrative process between the Breath of Life and Primary Respiration.

Long Tide- This movement originates from the field around us and travels up and down the mid-line of the body (the area just in front of the spinal cord along the vertebral bodies). Its rate is very slow - about 100 seconds for inhalation and 100 seconds on exhalation. This Tide corresponds to the bio-electric signals that come from the field which make contact with the tissues.

Dynamic Stillness – This is a place where the tissues can build potency and come into direct relation with the Original Blue Print and its origin the Primitive Streak. Where the tissues settle in *Deep Stillness* and potency can build to be taken later by the Tides out to the periphery. Motion Dynamic Stillness, feels like ground swelling and can even be felt as a sensation in the field as the body orients to health and integrates with the wider field of both the body and the environment around the client.

The Role of Fascia in the Craniosacral System

Fascial Dynamics

Fascia is the master communicator within all bodily systems. It is possible to sense all these layers of Tidal Movement coming from the rise and fall of Primary Respiration by the way it travels through fascia.

Fascia is the tough connective tissue which covers everything and connects everything in the body. This makes the body like one big sweater that is interconnected throughout. When one part is affected, the other parts will also be affected. This intelligent system of fascia is how Dr AT Stills was able to sense into all systems of the body by palpating. All systems of the body are connected through fascia.

The states of fluidity in the body are directly mirrored in the fascia system which acts like a living matrix. It's functional ability to shift and change, hold and support, and conduct, to fit the functional need of the body makes fascia a major contributor in the flow of information in the body.

Fascia is a continuum within the body and communicates throughout. (There is much intelligence in fascia.) Fascia is alive and full of fluid. Imagine how the earth changes shape with the pull of the Sun. Our bodies are like the Earth: our fluids are poly-rhythmic like the tides. Just as the earth reacts to the sun fascia reacts to the surrounding environment by how its fluidity manifests inside the body.

The Three Anatomies of Fascia

In essence, there are three anatomies of fascia, or states of fluidity found in the body which are identical to the three layers of the Tides. These terms were conceptualized by the originator of the Continuum Movement Theory, Emily Conrad, and have great likeness (or perhaps are identical) to the different layers of the movements present in Primary Respiration. Both concepts speak clearly about the fluid state of our bodies that is also reflected in fascia. Fascia is surprisingly full of fluid, and when looking at microscopically, resembles dew drops and spider webs, while also possessing the ability move and connect to other strands of fascia that are similar to neurotransmitters.

Cultural or Industrial Anatomy – Similar to the CRI and this anatomy relates to the state of our tissues under the stress of our modern daily lives. It tends to condense our tissues into a less fluid state, by literally narrowing our attention and bodies into a forward motion. In this state we are not very present in our back bodies; rather "speed up" in our nervous system anatomy (sympathetic nervous system dominant) in order to multi-task and navigate many types of information coming from various different directions.

Primordial Anatomy – Similar to the Mid-Tide, this anatomy relates to a slower pace in which we are able to integrate experiences from the past with experiences happening in the present moment. It is a state somewhere between the parasympathetic and sympathetic states of nervous system balance where the experience is relating to the whole.

Cosmic Anatomy – Similar to the Long Tide and possibly also Dynamic Stillness. It is a slower and spacious existence that is deeply connected to the consciousness of universal truth or spirit. It is within this state that all traumas can drop away and health can begin to re-surface into the tissue. The therapeutic process happens in stillness and the integration of health must be a gradual movement through the fluids of our tissues in a way that it can titrate as it spreads and moves along. It is like an integrative deep dive into unity where everything is simply connected and the source of complete restoration lives.

~

Not only is Primary Respiration the organizer of tissues operated by the Breath of Life, but it is also an aspect of a deep spiritual intelligence. Something emerges in Primary Respiration that is connected to source of life and is very much alive. It seeks to know itself and chooses to come into form, so the form can reflect its own original intention. Behind the understanding of how this system works, is the body's natural self correcting force which heals all injuries and traumas.

The long tidal movement of Primary Respiration originates from the field which is the environment surrounding the client all the way to the horizon. Primary Respiration moves in a fluctuating pattern of coming in and going back out like the tides, all the while organizing the tissues to create balance between its original intention, its experience and that which is in the present moment.

One of the most distinguishing features of the mechanics of Primary Respiration is its emphasis on the mid-line. The mid-line brings order and organization to the developing embryo as well as the adult. The way the embryo uses the Breath of Life and Primary Respiration to organize itself in utero is a morphological enactment of the exact way of how Primary Respiration and the Breath of Life operate and organize our tissues throughout the duration of life. It is through the study of the human embryo that we are able to understand the origin and intention of Primary Respiration. We can see a visible gesture of the invisible act of incarnation and realization, which the physiology of life continues to show every moment as we experience and move through consciousness.

Thus, the whole role of Craniosacral Therapy is to listen to these rhythms and to support the body in accessing its original health underneath all pain, trauma, illness, injury or disease. Craniosacral Therapists are able to be present enough in their own bodies so that they can listen with non-judgment to the layers within the clients' physiology that present for support. From a place of neutral listening, the therapist can witness how the body intelligence of the client can stimulate correction in the physiology and bring the system into balance at a speed that is exactly right for the client.

Chapter Four

Subtle Body and Soul

Clearly, there is a great intelligence behind what we can see. Our existence is simply a miracle. In Vedic teachings, the formation of the embryo is a metaphor for the expression of life. Spiritual embryologists also confirm that the dynamics of the embryo may be the only clear picture in which we can see these unseen realms interacting with matter. Consequently, the motions which are laid down in our formation as an embryo continue to operate within us until death. The process of death is physiologically epi-genetic and the same for *All Living Beings*. Depending on the species, the formation into existence is different for all beings. However, the level of the experience of formation on the conscious level is encoded into the fluid dynamics of the individual being. The unique circumstances in which spirit and matter interact create our own individual evolutionary process.

The Polarities of Embryological Formation

In Eastern culture the knowledge of the Subtle Body and the Soul are considered common and natural aspects of the reality of our existence. Vedic cosmology is a whole science of the Subtle Body, and its function and meaning of existence. The study of the subtle body is the study of spiritual physiology; or one could say it is the studying of a metaphysical map that guides us in our spiritual practice and delineates the pathways to higher consciousness.

The Subtle Body is the link between the gross (physical) body and the causal body (or abstract/spiritual body). It can be thought of as the bridge between the physical body and the divine principal in a human being AND in all living beings. Although it is invisible, it can be felt within the subtle movements in the fluidity of the Breath of Life in craniosacral therapy.

The Hindu understanding of these Subtle Body movements is illustrated in many ways, but is directly depicted through the meaning behind Nataraj or the 'Dancing Shiva' who represents (in this incarnation) the source of all life and dances the eternal rhythms of the cosmos. These eternal rhythms also move through all living tissues.

The Subtle Body pervades the entire physical body, giving strength and energy to its every action. It contains the seeds of every movement. Vedic cosmology contains the knowledge of the *living being* and of specific structures in the body that hold centers of energy from which life force flows. This brings consciousness into being at every level - including cellular - and allows consciousness to manifest as action. The gross body (physical body) is a manifestation of the subtle body, and the gross body carries out the movement or intention of the subtle body.

The body is the form of our soul. It is the movement of the soul that leads to our form and our existence in this world. The body is the vessel of expression for the soul. Soul is the motion and body is the form. It is the soul that forms the body. The closest thing we come to actually seeing this truth is in the form of the embryo. As an embryo, the primary act of the soul is to shape the body.

There is a great duality in the nature of our existence as humans. There is so much mystery underneath the presence of "I am" consciousness, which is unique to the degree in that only human beings appear to posses this quality. In the formation of the embryo, there are many phases of duality or polarity which it must go through in order to come into formation. Life is the great dance of duality between spirit, consciousness (mind), and matter. In the embryo, form is the final the actor and underneath its' meaning the "I am" consciousness is the orchestrator.

Vedic Understanding of the Invitation of Life and the Function of the Subtle Body

The pattern that grows in utero is the pattern that we take in life as human beings. What grows in utero contains the blueprint in life and every cell carries that pattern. The blueprint seems to speak a lot about the human condition and the orientation of our conscious mind. We live in a twofold body: in utero and, metaphorically, in the adult mind.

The Rig-Veda is the oldest existing spiritual scripture on earth. Its name, "Veda" means "the knowledge". It is regarded as one of the highest spiritual truths of which the human mind is capable. One of the systems of Vedic philosophy is based on a dualism involving the ultimate principles of soul and matter, called Sankhya philosophy. Sankhya is one of the six schools of classical Indian philosophy and is regarded as one of the oldest philosophical systems in India. A vast number of statements and materials presented in the ancient Vedic literature can be shown to agree with many modern scientific finds throughout all of science and psychology. It offers a unique understanding of the living sciences.

Within the study of Sankhya, there are 25 tattvas (realities) of creation. They are present at conception and also in the interactions we have with them for the rest of our lives. Sankhya philosophy regards the universe as originating in two realities: Purusha (universal consciousness or soul) and Prakriti (phenomenal realm of matter or the primal consciousness: consciousness known through the senses rather than through thought or intuition). They are the experience (Purusha) and the experienced (Prakriti). These two realities are at the root of the 25 tattvas; the tattvas are merely aspects of Purusha and Prakriti. In terms of Osteopathic studies, Purusha could be considered the Breath of Life itself and Prakriti could be the organizing force of Primary Respiration.

In Sankhya, Purusha is the "self" that provides the universe. It is also used to denote the masculine aspect of creation; the masculine quality being that of *universal consciousness.* In the Rig-Veda, Purusha is described as a primeval giant who is sacrificed by the gods so that all life can be born. The energy brings consciousness into matter so that it can be born and continue to evolve. Purusha is the subjective and active nature of the masculine in aspect *to* matter. Cosmic intelligence and universal truth come from Purusha. Another way to understand Purusha is that it is the part of the consciousness within the soul that is connected to whatever is universal consciousness.

Prakriti is the basic nature of intelligence by which the universe exists and functions through material existence. It is the "primal motive force" behind all that is living. It constitutes the universe required for absolute form to prevail and is at the basis of all activity in creation. Prakriti holds the nature of the feminine. It is the giver of life in aspect to spirit. Evolution comes from her, but Purusha and Prakriti work together. Prakriti also means nature. Nature described as environment and also the body constitution. Prakriti further divides animate and inanimate realms or more simply that which is enlivened and that which is lifeless.

Although these aspects are the beginning reflections of evolution coming into existence, they are not representative to a God and Goddess, but rather the beginning energies that first arise to building our consciousness. Purusha and Prakriti work together to form a more whole aspect called Mahat, the "I am" sense. Purusha separates out into countless Jivas or individual units of consciousness as souls which fuse into the mind and body of the animate branch of Prakriti. In Sankhya, the observation of interaction between mind and body is between the self (as Purusha) and matter (Prakriti). Together they create the "I am" (Mahat). These three energies (Purusha, Prakriti, Mahat), once realized, work within the three gunas or Aymakaras to bring us into physical existence.

The Aymakaras are the elements that allow self-identity or ego to be born. They are composed of the three gunas which are the tendencies or modes of operation known as sattva (creation), rajas (preservation), and tamas (destruction). The gunas are the cords that bind the soul to a flesh and self-identity.

In the ancient Vedic science of Ayurveda, the three gunas (sattva, rajas, and tamas) as they pertain to the human physiology are later in life called doshas: kapha, pitta, vata. The gunas are the properties of doshas and are *related to their functions in life*. The balance or imbalance of these doshas defines the Prakriti or nature of one's body. The gunas work in kinship with the doshas in the combination of the subtle body aspects and its interaction with the metabolic rate of the physical tissue.

The gunas were present in embryology and they always work together in all that is living through their transmutation into the doshas. They serve as the fundamental operating principles of Prakriti.

- <u>Sattva</u> is the 'energy of consciousness and knowledge' It embodies the fire (Tejas) and light. It is associated with the ayurvedic dosha Pitta and is affiliated with the formation and maintenance of the casual body or spirit body.

- <u>Rajas</u> guna is the 'energy of activity and the will to create'. It embodies the principle of movement in the wind dosha Vata and is associated with the formation into matter and maintenance of the subtle or energetic body.

- <u>Tamas</u> is the 'energy of stasis and matter'. It holds a micro-cosmic energy and the bio-electric field interact within the gross or physical body.

At conception, the three gunas are present in certain proportions and, it stays that way throughout life. They are constantly moving and will fluctuate between within a balanced state which is how we change. Their function, however, is always in a way of homeostasis.

At the formation moment of our birth, the condition of the doshas of the parents, the conditions of the constitution of the sexual act, the constitution of previous life, the quality of the egg and sperm all contribute to the first aspect of the nature and personality of our being. These constitutions are birthed in utero where it is wet, dark, and warm. During actual birth we enter an environment that is the total opposite, where it is dry, light, and cold. This type of adjustment is the epitome of the constant type of change in environment that our bodies and our doshas have to go through in order to keep health in the system. How we transition into environments at the birthing time also makes up a very specific constitutional presence of the doshas. How the doshas fall into balance between conception and birth gives the foundation of health from which to operate in life. These concepts are being realized in modern science today in the early 2000's with the evolutionary research coming that has come out of the genome project and tracking how experiences going on when babies are in utero and the birthing process can affect health conditions later on in life. Science has even linked the genetic understanding of how our grandparents' life experiences can affect health conditions in grandchildren.

To look even further into the three gunas as elements of intellect and consciousness we can also observe them in the mechanism of the subtle body present in Mahat the "I am" sense which is the development of prana or life force energy. Pure intelligence is pure consciousness. In Mahat the consciousness is always pure. The 'I' sense indicates duality, intellect and consciousness and are the same but they are also separate. We cannot say consciousness comes from intellect; consciousness is Purusha or part of the Breath of Life. However, we also need the energy to function through intellect. We also have airs that circulate through the different cavities of the body. They function to generate a life force to live and create the mind. These airs are called vayus and they circulate through the 5 cavities within our bodies at force measures and create the prana. Prana or Life Force gives us our intelligence and un-intelligence as well. The vayus are the energy that operates the physical substance within the human cavities in Tantric understanding of subtle body energy. In the universe, prana includes the forces of motion that keep the planets circling the suns. It would also be considered the essence of what drives the Breath of Life to move Primary Respiration. In the body prana is the life force or energy that is responsible for all the movement and activity, physical as well as mental. The prana is considered part of the subtle body. It is not a physical substance, but rather the subtle life energy that supports the gross body. In the body, the life force prana functions differently in the various areas of the body. To help facilitate movement of energy from one area to another in the physical body, the vayus operate in an overlapping way so that the Subtle Body airs can facilitate prana.

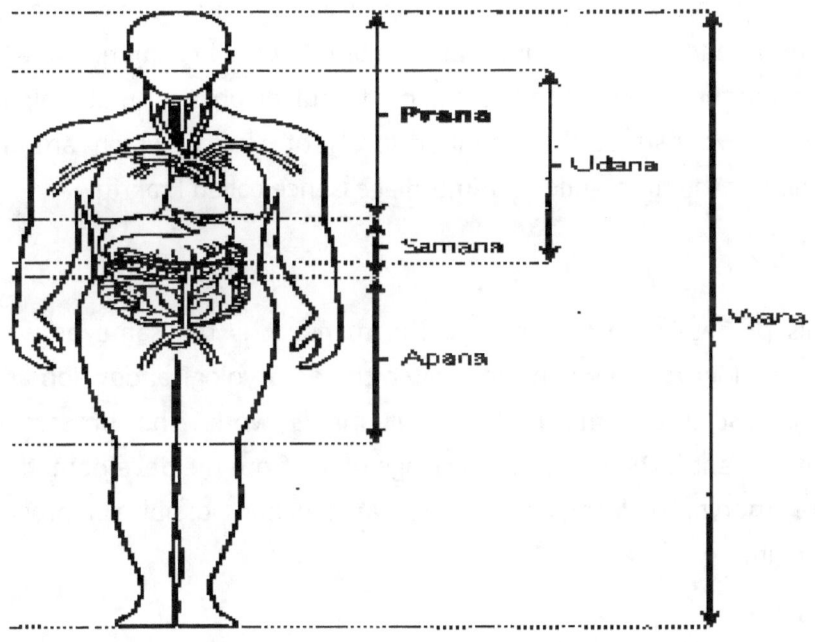

In the universe, everything evolves out of something. We do not come from nothing. Ornaments can be said to evolve out of metal. Pots can be said to evolve out of clay. Our world is filled with objects. Objects are made of compounds. Compounds are made of molecules. Molecules are made of atoms. Atoms are made of particles. Particles are made of subtler substratums. While one evolves out of the other, all of these levels of reality coexist and interact with one another.

Humans are also multi-leveled with the one level emerging out of the previous while each level still coexists and interacts with one another. This holds true with the physical development of our bodies in utero and also how our minds and brains work in conjunction with one another. While humans are made out of physical material, we are also constructed of subtler levels of reality, which are the products the un-manifest, primordial essence called Prakriti.

This process of evolution into the manifest is the same as what embryologists see when they watch the embryological develop and, it is also the same in how our minds work. The process of enfoldment is the same for any stage of life from the development of the embryo, too living and experiencing life, and possibly the process of dying.

Chapter Five

The Orientation of the Embryo

The Invitation on the Spiritual Plane - Before Conception

Creation is an invitation, an opening occurring between interactions somewhere in matter. Everything in existence is waiting for an opportunity. Stillness is potential and movement is manifestation. The potential for life is always present awaiting the right conditions and the opportunity to come into physical form. It has to wait for the moment where things on the spiritual side align with things on the physical plane.

Nothing in nature is forced. It is only man who forces through the complications of the mind. We are not the mere product of life. We are lifelong carriers of the Breath of Life. It is inherent in our nature to bring a biography into reality through the appearance of our lives.

Conception is merely a new development of life. Life never begins spontaneously. In the beginning our conception is the binding of the Breath of Life with matter. Death is the separation of these parts, and life is the appearance of soul.

The study of the embryo is perhaps a study metaphorically of how these two elements enact soul and matter. In the end we are not a product of our body especially when working with healing trauma. It is our biography that makes us who we are, and in order for the soul to experience life we must bring into appearance by means of our body.

Fertilization (The Gesture of the Seed)

One beginning phenomenal characteristic of the fertilization process has to do with the relationship between the sperm and the egg. It has been incorrectly taught throughout our culture that the sperm is responsible for fertilizing the egg. However, with a closer look, embryologists can see that this simply is not true. Fertilization is actually a process of polarization and the attraction between the oocyte and the sperm cell. Through a mysterious selection process the egg appears to actually choose a specific sperm by pulling the cell in. The act of fertilization is more than just the best sperm being the strongest and winning the punch into the egg. The oocyte allows the sperm to enter and together they fertilize. There must be some kind of attraction between the two cells in order for there to be successful seed formation.

The egg cells (oocytes) and sperm cells (spermatocytes) are polar opposites. The oocytes tend to specialize in a way that expresses the features and qualities of the cytoplasm of a normal cell. The spermatocytes, on the other hand exhibits the qualities and behaviors of the nucleus. The egg cell is very spacious and mostly filled with fluid while the sperm cell has very little space, not much fluid and is very condensed with nucleus type material. The egg cells moves very slow while, the sperm cells move very fast. The eggs cells are released one at a time while, the sperm cells are released by the millions. The egg cell lives in a warmer environment than the sperm cell.

Fertilization takes place when both the sperms and egg are at the end of their lives. If the will to create and the three gunas appear within the embryo, the gametes give their complete physical substance to fertilization. At this point the law of polarization shifts and begins a new phase of biological development that makes the embryo possible.

The *will to create* is what sparks the coming together of these energies, which can be directly seen within the first 24 days of conception and is the only driving force of our creation. It has nothing to do with genetics and DNA. It has to do with the true nature of things through the natural laws of fluid dynamics. The formation of living cells is generated by the interaction between soul and matter which is also responsible for the development of the gunas. In the fertilization process the gunas are formed by fluids dynamics as the Breath of Life makes contact with these elements. According to the Sankhya teaching there must be three elements of the subtle body present in order for life to move forth into realization:

Sattva - the energy of consciousness and matter.

Rajas - the energy of activity and the will to create.

Tamas - the energy of stasis and matter.

Without these elements there can be no possibility of seed formation.

The first week of embryology has the same characteristics of the seed of the plant. The "seed" is actually called the morula and is seed like when the components of the egg and the sperm come together.

Another fascinating understanding of the fertilization process is found in certain animals where morula (the fertilization product of the sperm and egg joined) actually acts very seed like. There is a phenomenon called Embryopause where the morula or "seed" interrupts its development at the stage just before implantation. In a deer, this occurs when the fertilization takes place outside of the spring rutting season. The morula is then stored in the womb "waiting" for the right time to implant. This embryopause also happens for kangaroos when the mother is still carrying a baby in her pouch. The seed will wait until the first baby has left the couch to implant. This ingenious intelligence that these animals' bodies have developed helps to insure successful survival for those species. In the case of human embryological development, this phenomenon has never been observed.

The first week of the embryonic phase just before implantation, results in the physical condition that merely offers the possibility for life to enter. It biologically takes the form very similar to a seed and even acts as a seed would in certain animals.

Center Out to Periphery Orientation (The Gesture of the Mineral)

Once conception is underway, the motion of the Breath of Life begins to differentiate the cell bodies in a way that is towards the periphery. *The first movement preformed is moving away from center to 'that which will be out there'.* This is a part of the duality of the human mind both being outside in periphery and inside. The embryo periphery goes out to feel around and is actually born out of the periphery first before coming into the center.

This process is the first example of how the human consciousness works and how the mind works in relation to the brain. The mind negotiates the outside world from the inside world, finds center then moves out to manifest its self into the outside world. We negotiate this process over and over again in life. It is also similar to the fluctuations of primary respiration which is the movement of our physiology throughout life. The long tide which is a very slow, long tidal movement seems to come from the field all around the body first, giving the inherent intelligence information that is relevant to its existence before traveling all the way up the energetic center of our bodies intrinsically organizing the physiology from the center outward. We start this differentiation as embryos and it continues throughout life.

The first movement of the embryo within this first week after conception is an expansion to confront what is out there. The physiological movement is from the center out. "Thus, the physical substance of the first week comes 'to life' in the same way minerals are alive." (Guus van der Bie, MD). Just as molecules and minerals grow out in all directions in layers from the center this phase of development gestures in the same way. We are born out of the periphery. The embryo goes out to feel around as its first motion of creating itself. After exploring the periphery and establishing what is out there the embryo begins the nesting phase which orientates the embryo to the dorsal and ventral polarity.

Dorsal Ventral orientation (gesture of germination)

Implantation begins during the first week of development. This is where the periphery cells begin to open up to become rooted and nesting begins.

The dorsal ventral aspect of our anatomical bodies comes from where we nest. Where we nest will be the back side. The umbilical cord roots to the mother on the back as if going back literally to feeling the mother. Psychologically, this gesture is the first element of feeling safe. The mother retreats biologically from the womb space to allow room for this new life and the mother and baby begin their silent 9 month dialogue of negotiating 'should we or shouldn't we'.

The embryonic sac of the placenta is also the consciousness of the embryo establishing separation. The embryo cannot exist without separation. The human mind cannot see, hear, experience without separation between the outer world and the inner. Thus, the gesture here begins the differentiation process of which will be pulled in toward the center. Conception and rooting as an embryo is so much more about dialogues between souls rather than simply biology, thus creating the magic present in our pure existence.

As we nest on the back side, the first appearance of the umbilical cord is called the connecting stalk at this early point in development. The amniotic sac is accompanied with a yolk sac and the area around them will be the placenta.

Caudal Cranial orientation (gesture of plant growth)

From the point of implantation, the cells of the newly conceived embryo begin to grow both upwards and downwards. By the end of the second week and into the third week, the embryo begins to show morphological and physiological features of a germinating and growing plant. The connecting stalk which roots the embryo migrates from what would be the back side of the body to the caudal or bottom area, symbolizing the actually roots of a tree. The Heart begins to appear at the area above the actual formation of the head, superior to the rest of the body symbolizing the head or branches of a tree. A mysterious Primitive Streak appears which gives an orientation as to where the central nervous system will develop while also indicating where the midline of the body will reside in the adult embryo. This Primitive Streak likewise symbolizes the body of a tree.

The physical substance of the second week comes to life in the same way plants are alive. This shape allows the foundational base for the vital organs and the body, as a whole, to lay down the Blue Print. The first major organs to appear are the Blood, Heart, and Primitive Streak.

The first major developments of the organs and their orientation to mid-line follow into the third week after conception. The mid-line or the beginning formation of the notochord will be the center of body and begins to form around 15 days after conception. The neural tube and notochord formation begins as a cleft like formation anatomically at the cleft associated with the bottom of the digestive system or rectal area. It follows up the pathway of the Primitive Streak from the bottom up while the Primitive Streak itself appears from the top down.

The Heart

The blood is the first organ to appear in utero. It first develops along the outside walls of the embryonic sac. Again, we see a pattern that starts on the periphery before coming into the center. The first movement in organ development starts on the outside before moving center to establish the area of the Heart. Blood, at this stage in development, moves to form blood vessels one cell at a time by clustering and then streaming. By cell metabolism, the blood moves purely to its own physiology without the presence of the Heart. Over time, the blood begins to find its way to center. After traveling along the periphery on both sides of the embryonic sac the blood meets on the superior aspect of the sac just opposite the connecting stalk and on the other side of the Primitive Streak (which is also developing at this point). By clustering and streaming it creates a place to which it will always return. This begins the development of the Heart. The formation of the Heart comes from the pathway of which the blood clusters and streams at this center point. A mysterious aspect of the Heart is that it is actually a ventricle. Ventricles operate by opening up their cavities to *receive* fluid than expels the fluid outward with their contractions. Due to this fact, there may be some question as to whether the blood actually forms the Heart or whether the Heart actually develops to house the meeting place of the blood.

On observation metaphorically the Heart becomes a place where we can become physically "I am". It is the first organized place in our anatomical formation that becomes a center point for our physical being. The Primitive Streak is also forming around this time(about 3 weeks after conception), but it is and always will be a mere streak of light of photonic matter referencing more to the energetic body then a tangible physical place that will be "I am".

The Heart is a very wonderful and mysterious organ. The Heart helps us to be upright like a tree in utero as well as a center place of which we can operate upright in the standing formation, which is unique to humans. It does this by viscerally bringing the spine upright as we begin to unfold in the third month in utero. The Heart is actually a ventrical. It opens to receive the blood then it expels the blood out. It begins anatomically over the head area and gives a point of reference for the soma to gather as a central location for the "I" am presence. It is also one of the three "brain" organs. The brain organs are organs of the body that have similar neurotransmitter substance and activity as the brain. All of the organs of the brain actually include the Heart and also the gut.

The growing inward actually does not start until the 3rd week. After the Heart is established on the cranial aspect, ectoderm comes together on the sacral (caudal) aspect down by the roots of the connecting stalk. The ectoderm (connective tissue of the embryo) begins to grow like a cave at the cleft of the backside and begins to transform into mesoderm (connective tissue of the embryo that will become the tissue of the nervous system). This mesoderm travels up along the backside of the remnants of the Primitive Streak and forms a staff. It is here in the embryonic stage that we begin to truly mirror the growth process of the plant life. The gesture is rooted down so that there is an extension upward. Growing out both ways from the center, just like a tree or plant.

Primitive Streak

As the blood forms and the area of the Heart is established the formation of the Primitive Streak instantly appears. The streak will be the center point for which the neural tube will form. The primitive streak is the original blueprint that lays down the foundation for the matter of what we will become. It is an energy line, literally a streak of light that becomes present within 21 days of our formation. As the cells multiply, which is the start of new life, this energetic Primitive Streak gives a middle point for the tissues to form which eventually becomes the mid-line of our physical body. The Primitive Streak also becomes a central pathway for the organizing presence of the Breath of Life and Primary Respiration which operate and organize along this streak throughout life.

Somewhere from the outside we gather to in towards the center along a mysterious Primitive Streak. The mechanics of its formation is scientifically unknown. No one knows where it comes from. However, science does identify its purpose, to create a center point of which we can form. Later, in embryonic development, the streak nearly vanishes. As adult embryos we still carry remnant cells within the vertebral disks in our spine making it a constant energetic line from which the Breath of Life can orientate. This place in the living human anatomy may be the same key place of which ancient Subtle Body studies out of India refer to as the Nadis.

In the ancient philosophy of Tantric yoga studies the Subtle Body is the pathway to the expansion of knowledge. The highest knowledge is the operation of the Subtle Body and is thought to the link 'the between places' of the gross (physical) body and the casual (I am consciousness or Mahat consciousness) body. There is reference of anatomy within this philosophy of the Subtle Body, called the Nadis.

The Nadis are anatomical points along various nerve pathways of which the prana or life force moves in a human being, giving it life and vitality to be here in this world. Prana is the life force that sustains the body and could be referring to what Osteopaths call the Breath of Life. Specifically speaking to the Primitive Streak, the Shushumna Nadi is a major center for life force that runs straight up and down the center of the spinal column and contains the five panch chakras (the chakras of the gross body or rather from the head down).

This is very interesting because from what Osteopaths have been able to see, the remnants of the Primitive Streak in the adult remain within the vertebral disks of the spinal cord. These two understandings, through the function of the Nadis in Vedic teachings and the function of the mid-line along the energetic remnants of the Primitive Streak in Embryology, may actually function as one and the same.

There is spiritual belief in the Osteopathic field that the Primitive Streak is where the Breath of Life enters the physical body, thus giving rise to form. However, it would seem by truly studying the jesters behind the entire embryonic formation that the Breath of Life was already present in the first moment of conception, when the egg cell allowed the passage of a specific sperm cell within her membrane and again when the multiplying cells grow out ward before coming in to form the actual body. The route of the Primitive

Streak does act as a passage way for the Subtle Body and is where transmutation takes place in the organization of the tissues in embryo. This transmutation process carries out its process through this route of the Subtle Body throughout the duration of life and becomes a center point for which the tissues organize themselves as the adult embryo integrates new experience in the tissues.

Folding in Orientation (Gesture of the Animal Kingdom)

In the beginning of the fourth week of development we begin the folding process. This is the true gesture of individuation and the true embryonic period. The neural tube closes and the gut tube which originates from the yolk sac moves upward and downward forming the entire digestive system by opening up the mouth and later (at 6 weeks) opening up the anus. In the fourth week the blue print is completely laid down for what we will become. This is portrayed by having a complete inner body of which we will continue to develop and grow throughout the length of life. There is now a vessel for which we can operate the inherent plan of the blue print and, the Breath of Life.

The gesture that begins the journey of individualization is seen as a sacred bow inward as the embryo is folding in towards itself. This motion is as if the being is making sacraments to what it will become, first by folding in towards the heart center of which is "I am". The heart folds in toward midline and assumes its place in the center of the body. The body then grows around the center of the heart. The developing arms eventually move outward to embracing this sacred organ. The legs will eventually grow around the umbilical cord symbolizing a root that will always connect us to other beings and the outside world metaphorically. The neural tube begins to fold into various creases that will be the different aspects of the brain, the creases being where the ventricles will be. The developing head also moves to rest itself at the top of the heart, right at the point where the pituitary gland will be developing.

In this folding process we additionally begin to mirror that of the four legged animal kingdom. To all the relations of this planet we will grow through their gestures, connecting us to all life, so we can become what will be.

Going Upright (Gesture of the Human Form)

The aspect of embryological development in the human embryo that distinguishes us from other beings of life comes when the embryo moves from being folded inward to the upright position. The motion of coming erect creates extremities. Extremities are ectodermal extensions of the metabolic system or rather the visceral/organ system. As the head comes up, the arms come out of the heart region. As the spine stretches upright the legs grow out of the gut region. In essence our arms are an extension of our hearts and our legs are an extension of our guts, which is so philosophical to the term following our gut. The extremities' grow out of the center metaphorically, similar to how our minds growing out beyond the center of which is our consciousness. Furthermore, the upper extremities' turn towards the sky and the lower extremities turn towards the earth connecting us to the spiritual planes of 'that which is above and that which is below'. The gesture of stretching and unfolding has to do with becoming freed from the inside.

In having to maintain the upright position the human being metaphorically becomes a creature of balance. "Only humans have a stable upright posture. The perfect rectangular relationship of the frontal, sagittal and horizontal planes in the human body is due to the persistence of the unfolding process of the vertebral column." This means that 'characterization of the process of the unfolding in and after the fourth week on the embryonic body becomes specific to humans". In opposition "animals considered close to human such as the apes or primates, have an unfolding process too." The difference is the "unfolding of apes and primates occurs in the brain, skull, and pelvic region but does not extend along the vertebral column." (Guus van der Bie, MD). Humans unfold along the entire length of the spinal column.

Epi-Genetics and DNA

We all start from this simple beginning of water dynamics, all relations of the earth from minerals, plants, animals and human beings. All life comes from water and it is movement that leads to its form. The water in the living form is an energetic representation of the essence in which the Breath of Life or the Subtle Body can travel.

Studies indicate that genes and DNA are organized by the fluid motion present in the embryo. They are not the organizers of human life. The role of DNA of the embryo sets up the basic mold or blue print of the nervous system. It is our experience that refines what we will become. But it is our experience that fills in the DNA.

The laws of nature do not change as we age. Healing and change in a human adult are guided by the same physiological principles as growth and development of the embryo. The embryo and the laws that govern are a potent symbol of life's vast potential, an archetype which is a literal example of the life forces that express themselves in the human form. "The processes of embryological development are guided by motion, relationships within the motion, metabolic fields, fluid dynamics, and a precision that is epi-genetic". (Blechshmidt (German embryologist). It is a process that is not dictated by genes but rather biology.

The earliest processes of human formation are not determined by genes but by these forces present within the fluids of the embryo. These fluid fields are expressions of the universal aspect stepping into consciousness. There is much insight into the study of genes that better indicate their role. "Genes are not self-emergent, but will operate when they are activated from outside signals such as presence or absence of nutrition, toxins, stress, emotions thoughts, and environmental signals."(Dr. Bruce Lipton based on his 13 year U.S. study called the Human Genome Project completed 2003). Based on this clearer understanding of genes it becomes apparent that the early formation of the embryo is driven solely by fluid dynamics!

Embryological Development and its Reference to Health

The principles of embryology and healing are all versions of the same force. If we are the continuation of the embryo, then the original pattern of our greatest intention always lays underneath the organic structures of the body.

What is even more fascinating is that these motions present in physiology present most powerfully in a mode of healing that is in the same formations of all the fluid dynamical movements presented in embryology. Not only are the embryological movements a gesture to the function of the human mind but also a real physiological movement that can present when our bodies move toward healing. Through the embryo we can see evidence of the matter by which mind and matter interact to create form. This is possible because of fluid dynamics and that we are made mostly of, water. "Water is the receptacle that receives spirit." (Masaru Emoto) "Water participates in the creation of the physical form in the embryo and then maintains the adult through its hydraulic, electrochemical, and spiritual power." (R. Paul Lee, DO)

In short, the Breath of Life or life force or Prana or 'Unconditional Love' is the very ground substance of all creation. The structural pattern of the life form exists in an energetic spiritual realm acting through the media of water. Our bodies are always working on a state of homeostasis and balance in the system no matter what presents. And it is within the still moments of our lives and within Primary Respiration that the system can transmute and allow the potency of our system to re-align toward a greater balance of health, than was before.

"The generative forces in the embryo are retained throughout life as healing forces. In the embryo, the morphogenetic fields direct the migration of tissue to organize the organism. In the adult, healing recapitulates the development process. Migration cells in the embryo establish the pattern for the movement of energy, and the delivery of water and nutrients. The removal of waste travels in the opposite direction. This to and fro motion is palpable. It represents the reciprocity described by Still." "With trauma, imperfection of the structural element displays imperfection of function. If we refer to the perfection of the original pattern, both structure and function resume their original perfection." "In the tissues, we palpate health as a full and systematic tide. Peace, harmony, and balance are the outward signs of health in the behavior and demeanor of the individual." (R. Paul Lee, DO)

The movements of Subtle Body energy of the Breath of Life and Primary Respiration brushes within matter at conception are the same that form our bodies completely, and their motions live with us in constant evolution until death. We are patterns of energy or fluid interacting with the outside patterns of energy or various forms and fluid patterns. Within consciousness, the physiological components, emotional components and mental components of the Breath of Life are in constant movement of coming in and going back out. Its intelligence is the same as what moves the mind and all of the inherent intentions behind action and various forms of health.

Chapter Six

Fascial Dynamics: How One Part Affects the Whole

There are two basic forces at work in the living body: the Biodynamic Potencies generated by what Osteopaths call the Breath of Life and Biokinetic or Conditional Forces introduced into the system via trauma and life experiences (inertial fulcrums).

Biodynamic Potency is the universal force behind the Breath of Life and is the inherent authority that maintains order, integrity and homeostatic balance. It manifests at the moment of conception, organizes cellular differentiation, embryological development and is with us throughout life. Potency manifests as a bioelectric biomagnetic field phenomenon and it is a unified field of health around which fluids, cells and tissues organize. This is an intelligent life force that maintains the order and coherency of the cellular-tissue field and

---

Important Natural Fulcrums

- Sutherland's Fulcrum : Membranes and Connective tissue (anterior end of Straight Sinus, just anterior to where the falx and tentorium meet)

- Sphenobasilar Junction: Bones

- Anterior wall of 3rd Ventricle : Fluids

- Lamina Terminalis : Central Nervous System (this is the tip of the embryological brain in the early weeks of development)

---

generates both fluid and tissue motility through the transmutation process which is carried out through Primary Respiration.

Biokinetic Forces are conditional patterns of restriction or trauma forces (also called inertial fulcrum as applied in Craniosacral Therapy.

Fulcrums are a still place around which motion is organized. There are two types of fulcrums that that can be found in the natural world. In reference to Biodynamic Craniosacral Therapy, **Natural Fulcrums** are places that organize the fluid and tissue world in our bodies maintain coherency of form and function.   And **Inertial Fulcrums** are *conditional forces* that reflect our life or experiences and they do not shift or move as easily in the phases of primary respiration.

Another area where natural fulcrums are found in the body is within the horizontal fibers of fascia. Most fascial sheath run **vertically** (up and down) but there are some locations in the body where there are dense collections of **horizontal** fibers (side to side) that act like a hoop to hold our structure up right as well as creating a frame work to hold our organs. *These are considered natural fulcrums of the fascial system.*

The 3 transverse/horizontal fascial sites on the torso
1.   Respiratory Diaphragm
2.   Pelvic Diaphragm
3.   Thoracic Diaphragm
4.   Hyoid Bone

Because of the location and purpose of these Horizontal/Transverse Diaphragms they tend to be subject to forming restrictions.

The Fluid Dynamic understanding behind Biodynamic Craniosacral Therapy is a particular approach into the study of the natural and creative forces that organize the human body. The forces that are found throughout the natural world are the same forces that we carry within your physiology. They include a subtle ordering principle that drives the creation, development and maintenance of all systems. Within the expression of these forces is a polyrhythmic movement that is stable and palpable, moving in cycles known as Primary Respiration. This movement is omnipresent in all living organisms and it moves in a natural expansion-contraction pattern that is very different than the respiratory breath and the heart beat. Interactions with the movements present in craniosacral understanding can have remarkable health benefits.

All organisms seek to find balance individually and within their whole ecosystem. We can see this clearly demonstrated in nature when we look at a tree that continues to live and grow by adapting its growth pattern around dismemberment or the way the tree may grow in a spiral around another neighboring tree that stands very close by. We also see how an ecosystem will strive to find balance when there has been damage or destruction by man, it adapts by producing imbalance in order to come back into balance. Our bodies work the same way. The manifestation of imbalance, disease, illness, and effects of mental health are all demonstrations of how our body seeks to find balance. We all carry this self corrective force within our bodies which are generated by deeper organized movements in the physiology and function as a continuum.

Inertial Fulcrums

Sites which have lost ability to shift within the inhalation and exhalation phases of primary respiration. *Organized resistance to movement*

They can be caused by:

* Physical or psychological trauma
* Injury
* Can come from as early as conception
* Early Childhood trauma
* Pathogens
* Toxins
* Environmental Issues
* Genetics
* Other forces overlaid on the natural organization of the system

Chapter Seven

Anatomy of the Autonomic Nervous System

As Craniosacral Therapists we work with the Blue Print of the self. A blue print that exists before trauma and injuries ensue. Our blue print is similar to the roots of a tree, always there always feeding and sustaining us. No matter what happens to us in our lives there is a fluid motion within us that is very much alive, yet it is deeply rooted into Stillness that is our blue print.

~

When we experience trauma it can get sealed off in the connective tissue. A ball of Life Force Energy literally becomes encapsulated within the system. As life goes on after trauma the connective tissue creates a shape or pattern that can eventually lead to pain or illness in the body. Biomechanical ways look at the shape and try to fix it. In Biodynamic ways we look at the health that is always there.

In order to understand where there is Health within the places that are suffering we must realize that all sources of suffering in the body either, physical, emotional or mental come from how our nervous systems are wired and how this system is relating to the experience. The Breath of Life interacts with the body and is the main living system that carries us through life and offers immense healing to those areas that are imbalanced, but NOT all imbalances should be perceived as something less than whole. The nervous system informs us every moment about the nature and safety in the world that surrounds us. How resourced the nervous system is will always be the determining factor as to whether the potency of the Breath of Life is able to move throughout the living body system.

Anatomy of the Autonomic Nervous System: *The Role of the Autonomic Nervous System in Craniosacral Theory and how it's Connected to the Whole Body through Fascia.*

Muscle memory is the strongest memory we carry in the body. When a movement is repeated over and over in the body, it creates a long term memory which eventually allows the movement to be performed without any conscious effort. This type of memory is essential to the performance of athletes who rely of repetitive training to ensure success during competitions. Most athletes will tell you that all the hard work of training seems to take over during their performance events, that they step out of any thought process all together and that the body literally takes over. Muscle Memory is not just about memory in the muscles but rather memories stored in the brain. It's a form of Procedural Memory that are encoded in the brain and when accessed are used without the need for conscious control or action. Think about what it was like to learn to tie your shoes when you were little. It took great effort to learn the basics, many sessions of failed attempts and trying to remember which loop goes through what. But eventually it just became second nature and most adults don't even think twice about how to do it.

Consequently, muscle memory plays a major role during injury. Your body, brain and muscles remember the actions the resulted in injury. Even after the muscles and tendons heal, the body will automatically contract anytime the body is positioned in a similar manner the initial injury occurred. This is why people experience the ghost pains and holdings in their bodies many years after injury occurs, and why old injuries come back to haunt us as we get older. This frustrating phenomenon can be very debilitating for many people who have experience injury.

This type of imprinting in the body creates strong neuro-pathways or, associations in the brain. Neuro-pathways can be compared to trail making in nature. The more you hike down a certain trail the more the trail will become more visible and easier to follow. If you decided to make a new trail it would take much effort in forging in the beginning but the more you consciously hike onto the new trail eventually it would become as easy to follow as the first trail, while the old trail would become overgrown and perhaps harder to even make out after some time. Our brain works the same way. The more we engage in certain activities the easier they become.

There is a different type of memory we carry in our bodies that is also an implicit. Implicit memories are previous experiences without ones conscious awareness and are not necessarily part of our waking consciousness. Specifically this type of memory can be directly related to the nervous system and it has to do with psychobiology of early childhood development and the maturation of the pre-frontal cortex and limbic structures which are based on reoccurring experienced with the caregiver.

Most of the major imprinting in between the sympathetic and the parasympathetic nervous system begins in the womb as the baby develops and continues until around 7 years old. While major wiring in the frontal lobe of the brain continues on into the late 20's (things like writing and complex cognitive tasks such as inhibition, high level functioning and attention) the bulk of our nervous system is wired earlier on.

Bonding involves the nervous system and it is through the bonding experience we are hardwired in the nervous system. Before birth the baby is very tuned into what the mother is experiencing and begins to form its nervous system wiring according to what the mother is bonding with in the outside world. Babies share all of mom's chemicals while in the womb. If mom is resources, happy and calm the baby builds a nervous system that will be parasympathetic dominant. If mom harbors unresolved traumatic elements, is malnourished and highly stressed during pregnancy, the baby will build a nervous system that is sympathetic dominant. When babies are born they rely completely on the physical, emotional and mental status of their caregivers. Babies are completely helpless until they can grow big enough to take care of themselves in the teenage years through adulthood. Attunement of Mom is the essential way to learn about the outside environment and, babys' experiences are being recorded into implicit memory about if the world is a safe nurturing environment, or if the world is a difficult place where comfort, attunement and the lack of basic needs are scarce. All this learning contributes to how the nervous system is wiring itself preparing the little one for the life ahead.

The unborn and infant child experiences what the mother experiences, what the family experiences, and builds their body to suit this environment – this provides the template for physical and mental health decades later. This premise is called attachment, which is a scientific word for the process of relationship that develops during pregnancy through age 7 years old. During this time in a persons' life (from conception to 7yrs) it is laying down the basic structure for relationships with self and others, coping with stress, physiological processes like cardiovascular, neuro-endrocine, respiratory, glucose regulation, and immune system functioning.

Unborn children can be so intimately wired from the beginning of development psychologically but also in relation to their lifetime health. For example, inhaling high amounts of traffic pollution causes utero epigenetic changes that increase the risk of developing asthma as a child and 4 times higher chance of developing cancer later.

Other possible altering prenatal experiences:

- Depression

- Previous Reproduction Loss

- Drug use including nicotine, alcohol

- Poor nutrition

- Domestic Violence

High Stress is a fact for many pregnant and new mothers' lives, rich and poor. Cortisol in high levels is toxic to the unborn and infant child – it reduces the number of cells in organs, nerve supply and blood supply, thereby making them vulnerable to disease processes later in life. 50% of chronic disease like heart disease, coronary artery disease, stroke, and osteoporosis are liked to prenatal in etiology. (Nathanielaz, '09 Gluckman & Hanson '04) Serious mental illness like bipolar disorder and other psychotic illness have up to 75% etiology in prenatal and early life attachment (if there is genetic vulnerability (genes will turn on according to circumstance) Daniel Siegel '09.

Moderate stress in small amounts is good for babies because want us to be able to develop strategies to take back control of our environment especially in the last trimester of pregnancy.

Strategies for Stress

- Tune In

- Talk to babies – they are listening, learning your voice, learning to talk by moving their bodies.

- Gain the appropriate weight, get folic acid, omegas, fruits, veggies, fish and organic if at all possible.

- Exercise: 30mins of moderate exercise daily (it makes you both smarter and less stressed).

Spending time tuning in is one of the best guidance tools we can encourage pregnant mother to do during pregnancy. By the 2nd half of Pregnancy babies are definitely open to direct communication. Studies prove that if mothers spend time in quiet stillness each day (up to three times a day up t0 50 minutes each time) they will begin to develop a strong sense of what their baby wants to communicate. They can even ask questions like, do we need this ultrasound? And get accurate answers. They also have an easier birth and postnatal period. *(From German Researcher Dr. Gerherd Schroth 2009)*

The state of the Autonomic Nervous system also reflected in the state of elasticity and fluid of the fascia. Studies have shown that chronic pain might not only be caused by physical injury but stress and emotional issues as well. People who have been diagnosed with PTSD (Post Traumatic Stress Disorder) have a higher risk of developing chronic pain. Hence, we can see that imprinting in the nervous system is very similar to the mechanics of muscle memeory and are directly related.

Here we will learn the mechanics of the nervous system and how it relates to the whole. There are **three branches of the autonomic nervous system***:*

Parasympathetic – The Rest and Rejuvenation portion of our nervous system. The parasympathetic branch of the nervous system regulates organ and gland function, the digestion process, and sleep. The main nerve that is responsible for regulating this entire system is the Vagus Nerve. **The Vagus Nerve** arises from the central nervous system and is the longest cranial nerve out of 12 cranial nerves that existent. *Note: Cranial Nerves are 12 nerves that emerge directly from the brain, in contrast to spinal nerves, and are a part of the Peripheral Nervous System. The purpose of the peripheral nervous system is to connect the central nervous system (or rather the central primitive parts of the brain) to limbs and organs.* The vagus nerve is also translated in to cranial nerve X (ten). Its name is derived from the Latin meaning of 'wandering' because is snakes around and reaches from the brainstem to innervate all the organs. It exits the skull from the jugular foramen, crosses underneath the collar bones and begins to wander around to all the viscera below the head, to the neck, chest where is exits into the abdomen through the muscular foramens of the diaphragm muscle to the abdomen.

Sympathetic Nervous System – The Fight or Flight portion of the nervous system and innervates almost every organ system while regulating the up-and-down mechanisms of adrenaline which helps the heart and body spring into action the moment danger enters into our field. Adrenaline causes the effect of fight or flight and includes increased heart rate, pupil dilation, increased blood pressure and increased sweating. It is a bit of a mystery as to how the sympathetic nerve bundles connect to the central nervous system considering it is not a cranial nerve and does not attach anywhere specific into the brain stem. However, it is a vital part of the Peripheral Nervous System. The Sympathetic Nerve fibers arise in the spinal cord by a mysterious synapse process reflectant in what is called the preganglionic motor neurons which acts something like a neuro-pathway that somehow conducts an electrical component. Motor Neurons carry signals from the spinal cord to the muscles in order to produce movement. These motor neurons pass into the **Sympathetic Ganglia Chain** which, are organized into two chains that run parallel to one another and on either side of the spinal column all the way down to the Ganglion of Impar which are the sympathetic ganglia chain rests into the front of the sacrum. These little nerve bundles, all along the sympathetic ganglion chain, are responsible for turning on and taking over the entire body in a moment's notice of danger or immediate threat.

Social Engagement Nervous System – Is a newly discovered aspect of the nervous system and is based on the Polyvagal Theory. This theory focues on the Ventral Vagal Portion of the Vagus Nerve and is considered to be the smart vagus because it is associated with the regulation of sympathetic nervous system using social methods such as facial expressions and social communication that could self sooth or calm the strong fight or flight response in ourselves and others. **The Ventral Vagal** portion of the vagus nerve develops later on in life and is a part of the social engagement nervous system. Its function is crucial in the bonding process, love, empathy, and intimate contact.

In case of a threat we will try the social engagement nervous system first by orienting to the situation and surrounds, communicating using eye contact and facial expressions. The social engagement nervous system helps to balance out the para-sympathetic and the sympathetic nervous systems when we are under distress. This theory also carries an understanding of Mirror Neurons. Mirror neurons are neurons in the brain that fire in the same patterns when both a person acts and when the same person observes the same action performed by another. These neurons help us to sync our brain waves and ways of thinking in order the share ideas. They assist us in learning skills and different ways of being by imitation and are important to understanding the actions of others. These mirror neurons are extremely important for babies who will focus very intently on their caregivers face and begin mimicking those facial expressions and learn how to adjust their facial expressions and actions to get what they need. These mirror neurons play a role in the whole body, are directly related to the ventral vagal function and help create a real sense of resonance between beings. When you walk next to another person you naturally fall into the same step together and when you sit next to a person your heart beats begin to synchronize to the same pulse.

~

During a traumatic event, the nervous system does into survival mode and the sympathetic nervous system which is responsible for our fight or flight mode sometimes has difficulty coming back to a normal relaxed mode and the parasympathetic nervous system balance. If the nervous system stays in survival mode, stress hormones such as cortisol are constantly being released, causing an increase of blood pressure and dis-regulated the blood sugar levels which contribute to the immune system's ability to heal. If a person has experienced trauma prior to a current trauma or injury those old implicit memories can potentially become triggered which can exacerbate the effects of newer trauma. Often physical pain functions to warn a person that there is still emotional work to be done, and can be a sign of unresolved trauma in the nervous system.

What we carry from our early childhood experiences greatly effects how we handle the world as adults. Traumatized people respond to stress very differently than other people do. Under pressure they may act and feel as if they are experiencing the initial trauma all over again. Psychology is recognizing that people who experience trauma as an adult who had a safe early childhood and were securely attached can experience a trauma during adulthood and have the natural skills to heal from that trauma over time. Whereas, people who endured early childhood traumas and ruptured attachment in some way can experience the same adult trauma and find themselves in a place where they almost cannot even emotionally and sometimes physically survive.

Signs of Restrictions, Activation and Holding held in the Body:

Pain

Speeding up

Holding Breath

Shallow Breathing

Trembling

Cold Extremities

Intense Heat

Dissociation

Numbing

Shock or Overwhelm

Confusion, Disorientation

Obsessive Thoughts

Need for Control, feeling out of Control

Fear, Helplessness, anxiety, anger

Anything Chronic

Signs of Releasing and Resource

Warmth

Expansion

Vibration

Therapeutic Pulse or Twitching

Broader Perspective

Relational

Connected

Relaxation

Softening

Spreading

Movement feeling more organized

Sense of fullness or filling

Sense of wholeness

Breath Changes (particularly Deep Breaths or Sighing)

Belly Gurgles (Borborygmus)

Chapter Eight

The Source Behind Craniosacral Therapy

Form comes out of motion. We see this when we look upon the earth and her geology. It was the motion of the water, contained within the boundaries of rivers and streams that molded the canyons. Motion of liquid lava formed the earth's mantle. The magma that resides underneath the lithosphere or crust of the earth constructs the movements associated with plate tectonics, including the formation of mountains. Wind and water mold the mountaintops and canyons into their unique formations.

We also see 'motion giving birthing to form' present in biology, the study of life and living systems. The metabolization, respiration, and division of cells work to build and unify the living organism. The fluid dynamics of cellular motion provides a watery impetus for the existence of spirit. The spark of life within a seed is born from the mysterious movement that fertilizes it and creates growth of a plant. On an even larger biological scale, all life works together to create motion in a cycle of life and death that interacts with the whole ecology and health of the planet. Without this cycle our actuality and the planet as a whole simply would not be.

To go even further into the science of quantum mysticism, the working together of life in the cycle of birth and death creates the possibility for the platform of the spirit. The Breath of Life is living motion that breathes a dynamic essence and fashions creation into physical form. With motion a great paradox exists that entails a majesty of dynamic stillness. Dynamic stillness is essential to creation and is there to witness all that exists and to watch divine creativity form life. The paradox lies between the dynamic stillness and the motion of the breath of life. This polarity is the basis for the spark into being.

The essence of how life organizes and expresses itself never changes in nature. All life is connected in terms of the fundamental makeup of what we are, what we become, and finally death. A mineral body keeps growing out until wind and water wear it away and dissolve the body, slowly, over time. A tree or plant keeps growing upwards towards the sky rooting down through the earth until wind knocks it down or somehow it dries up and dies. An animal body grows, ages and learns from instinct until death. A human body also grows, ages and learns until death but the process is not from instinct. The human specialty is for learning and reasoning. The mastery and capacity to put the learning and parts together in an evolutionary process, is what sets us apart.

All life is an expression of higher intelligence. While science offers some solutions into the inquiry of life and its existence, it has missed something very essential in its quest for understanding of the physical world. The study of Physics is an excellent example of the Cartesian mindset which has overrun the scientific fields. Physics, even though it is the science of matter/ energy and the laws that govern existence it does not consider existence as a whole. It is only interested in what can be proved empirically. It is not the actual study of living beings. To actually study and come to understand the true function of a living organism one has to understand soul, and soul cannot be put into a mathematical equation. All life is here to express something deeper, something profound that lies beneath.

To understand the science behind the living world one has to look openly and beyond the traditions of the scientific world. Fortunately, there is a clear shift happening in these scientific fields that is opening an acceptance of the greater mystery of that life and consciousness exists. Since 2003 Daniel Siegel a doctor of psychiatry has sought to redefine the definition of the mind. Together with the help of over 40 nuero-scientists, psychologists, psychiatrists, anthropologists and over a dozen other fields of science from around the world, he came up with a better understanding of the mind. They proposed that the mind is "a process that regulates the flow of energy and information" and "the mind uses the brain to create itself". This definition was contributed and in agreement with a combination of global cultural understanding, neuro understanding, psychological understandings and is cohesive to the laws of scientific understanding as well.

You may ask yourself, what does the understanding of consciousness and the mind have anything to do with the mechanics of how motion creates form? In the field of American Psychology even the concept of consciousness has been taboo because it is so elusive. However, "consciousness is important to the central understanding of biological life just as much as the laws of gravity." (Francis Crick Nobel Prize-winner for his co-discovery of the DNA double helix)

On a broader perspective in the western field of psychology and neuroscience, 'the brain produces the mind' is still currently the mainstream stance of psychiatry, but the mind is so much more than the brain. Neuroscientists' believe that the mind is just the activity of the brain. However, this kind of information is only part of the story. Again like all the other forms of science, Neuroscientists' are speaking only from what they can see. "The view that the mind is only the activity of the brain is only part of the story. If fact the mind not only can use the brain to create itself, but it can actually change the structure of the brain." (Daniel Siegel)

The mind is made up of more than just thoughts and images. The mind is also made up of feelings, emotions, and sensations in the body. The brain is the neuropathology for the neuro connections throughout the brain tissues in the skull. However, the brain also entails the whole nervous system and visceral system. Firing of neuro-pathways is proven to happen all over the body, not just in the organ of the brain. In essence, the brain is actually the whole body! It is the mechanism for energy and information flow. The energy and information (the mind) flows through these neuro-connections. The mind is the way we organize.

The triangle of well being in a human entails how we share energy and information flow between all the systems and tissues of the body. The brain is the vessel of the mind. The mind is the driving force behind organization but not only for the tissues. Again we come across another paradox, for the mind also is the organizing principle behind the play of memory and relationships between each other. This creates a polarity that moves from an organizational force to regulatory force that finds equilibrium between the internal and external worlds. The way we share energy and information between each other forms the bases for relationships. The mind is a regulating process, the brain is the mechanism of how it flows, and relationships are how we share that.

Obviously, there is a great Intelligence behind what we can see. Our existence is simply a miracle. In Vedic teachings, the formation of the embryo is the metaphor behind the expression of life. Spiritual embryologists also confirm that the dynamics of the embryo may be the only clear picture in which we can see these unseen realms interacting with matter. Consequently, the motions which are laid down in our formation as an embryo continue to operate within us until death. The process of death is physiologically epi-genetic, and the same for *All Living Beings*. Depending on the species the formation into existence is different for all. However, the level of the experience on the conscious level is encoded into the fluid dynamics of the individual being.   The unique circumstances of which spirit and matter interact create our own individual evolution process.

The Main Objective of Craniosacral Therapy:

Is to find restrictions and/or compressions (inertial fulcrums) in the fascial system and cranial vault which are caused by injury or trauma AND could cause dysfunction/disease in the body (possibly effecting other systems then where the initial inertia manifested) if left untreated. The main objective of this work is to support and listen to the body in a way that honors the body's natural ability to always be in a state of balance, even in the face of disease, illness and chronic pain. Our job as practitioners of this work is to support the health, listen to the body from a neutral non-judging way while supporting the stories and patterns that are there in the tissue to settle, soften and resolve just as it's ready to do so on its own. We augment this by knowing the anatomy, Being in our Body with a wide open listening field, very present with the client in a safe Relational Field (one that is not diagnosing, giving advice or even stating what we hear in the system at all, but merely reflecting). We don't actual DO anything except listen and offer contact with Floating Hands. In this way the tissues organized around restrictions and compressions have a chance to release, thus affecting the whole body/mind system.

Chapter Nine

Anatomical and Physiological Realms: The Nervous System Tissue and its Relationships to the Primary Respiratory Mechanism

~

The Meninges

The Central Nervous System is a vital system to our health and its main operating system lives in the very center of the brain. This system is very delicate and needs to be protected. There are several layers of tissue that surround and protect the central nervous system. Part of the protection is provided by the Meninges the other part that protects is the Cerebral Spinal Fluid (CSF).

The meninges are the membranes surrounding the brain and spinal cord. They consist of 3 layers:

- **Pia Mater** – is the delicate innermost layer of the meninges and means tender mother in Latin. In hugs the very closely to the outside of the cerebrum (physical tissue of the brain)
- **Subarachnoid Space** – This is a layer of fluid (not an actual meningeal layer) that rests between the Pia Mater and Arachnoid Mater. *See section below*
- **Arachnoid Mater** – means 'spider like mother'
- **Dura Mater** – means 'tough mother' and is the outermost layer and is attached to the bone.

Subarachnoid Space and Ventricles

These layers surround the brain and spinal cord providing protection, stability and house the shock absorbing Cerebral Spinal Fluid (CSF).

- Between the Pia and Arachnoid Mater is a fluid filled space called the **Subarachnoid Space,** which is where the CSF circulates.
- Within the subarachnoid space of the Meningeal system are pockets deep in the brain that are like cisterns (something liken to water bags) called **Ventricles.**
- *Ventricles* are where CSF is produced via the *choroid plexuses* and the *subarachnoid space* is where the CSF circulates around the brain and spinal cord.
- We have *4 Ventricles in the brain and one lumber cistern* (which does not actually produce CSF but is a water sac similar to the ventricles and is located around L2). The lumbar cistern houses the cauda equine (the horse tail branches of spinal nerves that run down the leg).

Ventricles

There are four spaces filled with CSF located in the center of the brain that, act a little like water bags to protect the cerebrum by supporting and cushioning its weight. All the ventricles contain choroid plexuses which produce cerebral spinal fluid by somehow filtering and allowing certain elements of blood to enter into the ventricles.

Two Lateral Ventricles – These ventricles lengthen across a large portion of the brain. The anterior aspect of these water bags are located in the frontal lobes, extend posterior into the parietal lobes with the inferior horns found in the temporal lobes.

Third Ventricle – The third ventricle is located between and slightly below the two lateral ventricles. It is nestled in the center of the thalamus structures and hypothalamus on either side. The thalamus is a pair of oval shaped organs that send out messages regarding sensation. The hypothalamus is an area below the thalamus and it is important for temperature control, appetite and sleep.

Fourth Ventricle – Located between the cerebellum and the pons.

Together these ventricles resemble something similar to a bird and even moves with the pumping of CSF and the motion of the tides like a bird taking flight:

Inhalation or filling of the CSF: head down (beak of the third ventricle), tail rises (horns of the lateral ventricle) and wings spread (lateral ventricles fill).

Exhalation squeezing motion of the CSF: the whole body narrows like a bird taking flight with the beak of the third ventricle moving up slightly.

Reciprocal Tension Membranes

They divide and support the hemispheres of the brain via Reciprocal Tension Membranes (RTM).

*   **Falx Cerebri** – separates the Right and Left Hemispheres of the brain. Attaches to crista galli aspect of the Ephmoid Bone and follows along the Sagittal Suture to the foramen magnum of the Occipital Bone.
*   **Tentorium Cerebelli** – Supports the weight of the brain and suspends it above brain stem. Attaches to sphenoid anteriorly extending around via temporal and parietals.
*   These 2 sheaths attach together at Sutherland Fulcrum.

Dural Tube

*   The meninges of the brain come together at the Foramen Magnum (C2-C3) where they fall inferiorly (downward) freely floating all the way down to the lower vertebrae (L1) and the sacrum where it attaches again before branching down into many nerves that flow out like a horses tail (cauda equine) down through the lower lumbar and sacrum to innervate the legs.
*   **Dural Tube** – The relationship between the cranial vault and the sacrum is called the Dural Tube. It creates a physical and energetic space between the occiput and the sacrum. Spinal nerves also exit through the Dura as they extend distally in the body.

~

Cerebrospinal Fluid

Cerebral Spinal Fluid is a relatively clear fluid produced within the Ventricles of the brain, via the Choroid Plexuses. We hold approximately 150ml of CSF. This fluid is contained mostly within the membranes around the Brain and Central Nervous System but also surround the parameter of the spinal cord as well as within the central canal of the spinal cord itself. The total volume is replaced, produced and reabsorbed every 3-4 hours. The purpose of the CSF is to:

- Cushion, nourish and protects the brain and spinal cord – water beds act as shock absorbers
- Buoyancy: reduces the weight of brain from 1500 gm to 50gm, reducing the pressure on base of the brain
- Excretion of waste products: by its one way flow of CSF to the blood
- Transports hormones from one part of the brain to another
- Carries Potency or 'Liquid Light' and Moves like a tide like motion.

The Vital Intelligence of the Breath of Life is expressed through the cerebrospinal fluid which lays beneath the anatomical structures of the brain and nervous system. 'The cerebrospinal fluid is the highest known element within the human body.'(Michael Kern) It contains the life force energy that is the 'vital intelligence' for our entire being. Cerebrospinal fluid is the communicator between the intelligence of the Breath of Life, the central nervous system and the entire body. This intelligence of the Breath of Life drives even the respiratory breath and the heart beat. The potent life force energy given by the Breath of Life is the invisible element found within the cerebrospinal fluid. This intelligence literally speaks to every cell in the body and gives us a means to exist. It is a potency manifest at the time of conception, in the form of intention. The vital intelligence of the cerebrospinal fluid is essential for the proper functioning of our inherent health.

There is a basic law in science that states movement equals life. The expression of this 'life force energy' comes in the form of movement. There is a tidal force that comes from the field through the long tide, moves along the remnants of the primitive streak or energetic midline present in the vertebral discs of the spine, and somehow percolates into the cerebrospinal fluid then extends out through the nerves into the fascial system.

The movement of the cerebrospinal fluid mirrors the exact movement of primary respiration present in all the tidal bodies and cellular respiration. It synchronizes with all body systems through motility.

How these Structures take on the Movements of Primary Respiration

- On a tissue and fluid level movement, the Primary Respiratory Mechanism is organized and defined by the cerebrospinal fluid which surrounds the brain and spinal cord.

- The meningeal system is the outmost surrounding layer of the central nervous system and is relatively tough and elastic. They protect the brain and spinal cord tissue.
- The movement of the PRM and the Breath of Life builds a Potency within the body: 1st along the remnants of the primitive streak present in the vertebral discs of the spine 2nd within the cerebrospinal fluid than 3rd ripples out to includes all the structures found within the body through nerve endings into the fascial system.
- The boney structures of the body move with both the movement along the energetic mid-line and the rocking of the cerebrospinal fluid in the cranium thus making the movement of the ventricles a natural fulcrum of all bones in the body.
- All the structures of the nervous system tissue mirror and record the experiences of life, which is reflectant in the actual feel of the meningeal system.

Venous Sinuses

- A connected one way highway of channels, that act similar to veins but are slightly different because they are literally cavities within the Dura, lacks any kind of valve typically found in veins and also is missing some of the traditional set of vessel layers typically characteristic of veins and arteries. The function of the venous sinuses system is to filter out old CSF and blood (after it has lost its potency) from the brain and spinal cord and brings it back to the Heart to be recycled.

- Arachnoid Granulations – Are little protrusions between the arachnoid and the pia mater that somehow takes the used CSF into the venous sinuses to mix with blood and it is carried back to the Heart via Jugular vein.
- Congestion in this system can lead to weaker immunity, headaches, congestion, fogginess, fatigue and low feeling of potency in the system.
- There is some evidence that this system also filters out chemicals from medications, anesthesia, as well as natural chemicals and hormones produced by the brain. Sometimes residue from these chemicals can take days to even years to process out of the brain. Supporting this system can be very beneficial for those who are having a hard time physiologically processing medication.

Why the Cranial Bones and Important to the Craniosacral System.

It is the movement of the cerebrospinal fluid that creates a microscopic movement of articulation between the cranial bones. When we are born, the bones of the skull are very soft and flexible, with very wide gaps in between the plates. The gaps between the cranial plates are called fontanelles and they are the very soft spots on a baby's head. This is so a baby's head can squeeze and mold through the narrow birth canal of the mother. The action of squeezing through the birth canal is important so that the baby can discharge embryonic fluid, from the ventricles through the ears, nose and the lungs. It is an important process that helps facilitate health in the nervous system and to begins the essential ignition process of potency that happens in the ventricles as CSF enters for the first time following birth, after the embryonic fluid is squeezed out and cerebrospinal fluid begins in work of potenizing the entire system. After birth as we gown the cranial bones also grow to fill in the fontanelles. However, because of the constant movement and pumping of the cerebrospinal fluid is present throughout our lives the cranial bones do not completely fuse together. There are varying degrees of miron movements present between the cranial bones to accommodate for cerebrospinal movement. The places where the bones join are called sutures.

The CSF moves the meningeal system and the RTM which are attached to the cranial bones. The CSF also moves up and down the spine within the dural tube all being driven by the pumping action of the ventricles. This is how the articulation of the cranial bones and the sacrum can give the practitioner clues to what is being held in the Fascial System via the meninges, dural tube, nerve endings and central nervous system.

The cranial bones, spinal column and sacrum are an important part of the craniosacral system. They serve as handles to what is going on underneath. Their movement or lack of movement indicates where dysfunction lies. Compression or injury to the bones can adversely affect the underlying structures of the system and vice verse compression or injury anywhere in the body can affect the structures of the cranial vault.

Motility – a biological term that describes the ability to move independently and spontaneously consuming or moving energy in the process. In the osteopathic understanding of the living organism, motility is described as all the movements in the body in relation to the CST movements, organ and nervous system movements. They are the movements best described at the rest and digest phase of the parasympathetic nervous system. Motility of the cranial bones is in direct relation to primary respiration via the tides, cellular respiration and the pumping to the CSF.

Motility of the Dural Tube: Flexion and Extension

- **Flexion/Inhalation and Extension/Exhalation of the Cranial Vault**
  - **Flexion** – Also called Inhalation = Fat head, occiput widening downward, sacrum also widening downward, limbs rotate externally, fluid in out body swells and widens.
  - **Extension** – Also called Exhalation = Skinny Head, Occiput narrowing upward, sacrum also narrowing upward, limbs rotate internally, fluid in the body narrows and the body curls inward slightly.

- **Inhalation**

- On inhalation as the cranium expands the occiput and the sacrum move downwards shortening the spinal cord pushing C.S.F. upwards.

- **<u>Exhalation</u>**

- **On exhalation the occiput and sacrum move upwards lengthening the cord and pushing the C.S.F. downwards.**

The motility of the cranial vault and spinal cord will mirror the movements of the full body Tides. There are many possibilities of rate within motility. The movement can be very fast as in the cranial rhythmic impulse (CRI), to a more integrated even lateral and/or medial type movement of the mid-tide, long full body movements of long tide and even dynamic stillness at times. Primary Respiration within the whole fascial system and the motility of the cranial vault are one and the same. This is how a craniosacral practitioner can treat anywhere on the body.

Listening with Feeling, Seeing, Knowing Hands as the Practitioner Settles into a quite place deep inside of Mid-line and into Stillness:
The 4 Characteristics of the Cranial Rhythm:
- **Symmetry-** Left to Right
- **Quality** – Strength
- **Amplitude** – away and towards mid-line
- **Rate** – How fast or slow

Anatomy of the Bones

o **Overview the Anatomy of the Sutures:** The sutures of the cranium are sites where tiny amounts of movement occur from the pumping and movement of the cerebral spinal fluid. These are the sites where complete fusion between bones never occurs do to the pumping of fluid underneath. Some important sutures to know are:

a. **Sagittal Suture** – along the parietals on top of the head in the middle.

b. **Coronal Suture** – Along the Parietals and the Frontals.

c. **Squamosal Suture** – Along the Parietals and the Temporals.

d. **Lambdoid Suture** – Along the Occiput and Parietals.

e. **Squamosal Suture** – Along the Parietal, Sphenoid and Temporal regions.

f. **Metopic Suture** – Along Frontal and Sphenoid region.

- **Occiput** – is actually 4 bones when we are born. This bone is in direct relationship with the fourth ventricle which is fairly narrow by nature. Contact of the Occiput can greatly relieve any compression to this ventricle and help to replenish the whole nervous system and help to spread potency manifest between all the tidal layers. The bone is also in direct relation to the optic nerve which attached to the pons near the back of the brain. Support here can also assist in balancing any literal compression on the pons, which is the site where all 12 cranial nerves attach to the brain stem. Superficially, the occiputal bone is where many of the neck muscles attach and support here can help to release and soften those muscles and help to decrease tension headaches. The junction between occiput and the temporal bone at the jugular foramen is where the vagus nerve exits the brain and this nerve. People who suffer from whiplash can greatly benefit with the practitioner working with this bone to both sooth any chronic tension in the muscles of the neck and to also help settle any nerve damage to the vagus nerve. In inhalation the occiput rocks inferiorly toward the sacrum and exhalation it rocks superiorly towards midline away from the sacrum.

- **Sphenoid** – Actually in 3 bones when we are born. This bone sits in the very center of the skull, behind the eyes, and the greater wings of the sphenoid are just at the soft spot at the temples. Many of the cranial nerves pass through various foramens present within and around this bone to innervate the eyes. . In a way, the sphenoid is the gateway for the nerves from the brain stem to the outside world as they pass through the Dura, through the sphenoid to innervate the eyes, ears and nose. Within the Dura the sphenoid holds the Pituitary Gland which sits in the Sella Turcica (Turkish saddle) which is a saddle shaped depression in the posterior portion of the Sphenoid Bone.

Together these two bones (Occiput and Sphenoid) create a natural fulcrum of how all the cranial bones articulate. The meeting place of which these bones make contact is called the Sphenoid-Basilar Junction (SBJ). These bones (the Occiput and the Sphenoid) are actually considered to be the first two vertebrae, in Chiropractic work. That is because the balance of these bones effect all the articulation on the spinal cord below and any imbalance here can cause imbalance in overall health.

- **Frontal** – The Frontal Bone is in 2 pieces at birth and is fused together by the 8th year. This bone is in direct relation to the Pre-

Frontal Cortex which regulates cognitive behavior, personality expressions, decision making, and moderating social behavior. Differentiation is a skill that is developed here in the frontal lobe: things like managing conflicting thoughts, determining between good, bad, better, best, same and different. Cognitively matching: future consequences with current activities, goal making, and social "control" (the ability to suppress urges that, if not suppressed, could lead to socially unacceptable outcomes). This area of the brain also rests for a time on to the actual organ of the heart in embryology which connects its function to also listening to the messages of the heart. Support on this bone can help integrate a persons awareness of what is happening in their physical body as well as re-connect them to the messages of their hearts. This is also a site where the Falx attaches and decompression here can assist in decompressing the whole dural tube down the spine.

- **Temporals** - are in direct relation to the little bones and structures of the ear and to the Tentorium aspect of the Dura (the portion that devides the left and the right hemispheres of the cerebrum. These are the bones that Dr William Sutherland studied in his anatomy class that got him thinking that perhaps they moved similar to the fish gills because they sort of look like the gills of a fish!

- **Mandible** - is also known as the Jaw bone. It is in 2 pieces at birth. It is innervated by much of the various branches of Cranial nerve seven: the Facial nerve; making it a very important bone in relation to the social engagement nervous system.

The meeting place of the Mandible and Temporal bones are a site called the **TMJ** (Temporomandibular Joint and there are many issues that could arise here: pain, swelling, clicking, popping, limited range of motion, headaches, Neck pain, difficulty chewing or swallowing, difficulty breastfeeding for new borns due to birth trauma or even gentle births. Working with these two bones can greatly relieve any compression to the social engagement nervous system and conditions related to the TMJ.

- **Parietal** – The sutures on the top of the head is the opening of the crown chakra (the gateway to god). It is where we can transcend the need for material fixations that create judgment and discontent. The Centrum is directly below the crown chakra between the hippocampi which actually works as an antenna to the higher spirit and had direct visceral connections to the heart and to the sacrum because is in direct line anatomically with the two. The Centrum is the center line between the 2 hemispheres of the brain. The Temporalis muscles located on the side of the head and are part of the TMJ system can pull on the parietals and possibly cause ear pain. This bone has a relation to the venous sinuses because a long venous sinus cavity runs along the top of the head just underneath the Sagittal suture called the superior Sagittal sinus. Sometimes when clients are experiencing a lot of congestion within their venous sinus system they will complain of a lot of pressure along the top of the head.

- **Zygoma** - are also known as the cheek bones or the zygomatic processes. These bones are also important to the social engagement system because a portion of the facial nerve passes behind this bone. This bone can also help clients to integrate expereince both within their bodies and within the outside world.

- **Maxilla** - is in physical relation to the sphenoid, the frontal bone and the zygomatic processes of which it is behind. In the maxilla there is a deep sinus cavity which can be painful when they are full due to pressure or sometimes the pain radiates to the check bones (Zygoma bones). This bone includes part of the palate inside the mouth and can sometimes be the counterpart to what maybe compressing the whole craniosacral system due to its articulation with the sphenoid bone. People who experience migraines often have issues related to this bone. Anyone who has ever had extensive dental work many experience lesion patterns with this bone. Old issues around nursing can and attachment can mirror in this bone. Often children that suck their thumbs maybe subconsciously trying to decompress and articulation of the cranial bones due to birth. Breast feeding also helps to decompress the entire cranial vault after birth and coupled with warm responsive skin to skin contact with mother, with the freedom to experience the sleep wake cycle so present with babies can correct any amount of minor birth trauma experiences during the journey of birth. If babies do not get to have this opportunity and instead are somehow taken away from the mother and there is nor breastfeeding and a lot of poking and prodding by the medical team, this can record unsettling experiences about the world within the nervous system and at the same time stunt the de-compression that needs to happen for healthy brain function. The same is also true for C-section babies, breastfeeding also can help to naturally drain out all the embryonic fluid (whatever is left behind after the medical team suctions) and to also help in the ignition phase. All these experiences around breastfeeding, birth, suctioning, resource and trauma can all get recorded in how the bones of the cranium articulate (remember these bones are handles of what are going on underneath) and can specifically relate to the maxilla. This bone also holds the upper teeth and forms the inferior wall of the orbital cavity. Hence dental issues and eye pain can be helped by working with this bone.

- **Ephmoid** – Top of the Fountain Spray in reference to the Breath of Life. It also articulates with the pituitary gland via its close approximation from the Sella Turcica. It also relates quite directly with the remnant cells of the noto-cord via the lamina terminalis. It also is the site that attaches to dorsal end of the Falx Tentorium at the christa galli. This bone is spongy at birth allowing it to compress as needed. Completely ossifies by age 2. This bone is known to respond to electromagnetic fields and is believed to be involved in homing & orientating in birds, bees, dolphins, whales, salmon, trout, salamanders and bacteria. Other mystical understanding with this bone entail: Prana (the life force energy in the yogic and Vedic traditions) pick up from air, the relation to the 3rd eye which is the gateway to the soul and a place where energies of the outside world (air) meet life force within the body. This bone is in direct relation physically to the sphenoid bone and the entire SBJ.

- **Sacrum -** is not actually a cranial bone but it can mirror the articulation of the cranial bones by its connection with the dural tube. The dural tube is the free floating Dural like membrane (wrapping around the actual spinal cord) within the bones of the vertebrae that is a direct extension of the Falx and Tentorium. The Dural tube is attached to bone at C3 and L1 and free floating in between. It has been observed in craniosacral that the pelvis mirrors the articulation of the cranial bones due to the movement of primary respiration in the sacrum. This bone is actually 5 bones when we are born. The sacrum is thought to be associated with the root chakra and certainly holds a very metaphysical sacred element when balanced. Due to its articulation with the pelvis, working with this bone can bring great relief to the Sacroiliac joints (SI joints). The piriformis muscle (one of the major muscles in a group of 10 muscles that make up the pelvis floor) is also attached to the sacrum. The sciatic nerve passes through this muscle that is also attached to the sacrum, hence support on the sacrum can also help the release the piriformis muscle. At the bottom of the sacrum is a little extension that looks similar to a tail and this is called the coccyx. The coccyx, even though it is physically attached to the sacrum it is fairly free floating and is 4 separate bones at birth. The distal end of the sympathetic ganglia chain rests in the seat of the sacrum and the coccyx represents the very bottom of the sympathetic ganglion. The ganglion that bundle here the circuits that are ready to take over in a situation that would require us to run for or lives. Working in this area in a settled way could greatly help the sympathetic nervous system settle and slow. The motility in this bone mirrors the movement of the occiput. It rocks inferiorly towards the heels on inhalation and rocks superiorly toward the occiput on exhalation.

- **Vomer** - is a singlely paired bone located at the top of the palate between the maxilla at the mid-sagittal line and articulated with the ephmiod, sphenoid, palantine bones and maxilla. It is just a thin sliver of a bone but it can get jammed into the Ephmoid and effect the articulation of the SBJ greatly. This bone may too be related to nursing and attachment issues surrounding the nursing years.

- **Palatine** bones are a part of the nasal cavity and rest between the maxilla and the pterygoid process of the sphenoid. They are in the deepest portion of the palate on the roof of the mouth, just before the soft palate in the mouth. A portion of these bones make up the floor of the orbit.

Chapter Ten

Cranial Nerves

Cranial Nerve 1
Olfactory Nerve

Function: Carries the special sense of smell. This nerve is a special sensory nerve. (Special sensory nerves perceives smell, vision, taste, hearing, and balance.)

The olfactory nerve is the shortest of the twelve cranial nerves and only one of two cranial nerves (the other being the optic nerve) that do not join with the brainstem but, rather attaches directly to the amygdala (an almond like structure in the brain that is a part of the limbic system and plays a role in processing emotions). The amygdale is located within the cortex of the frontal lobe and just above the tip of the inferior horn of the lateral ventricle making this nerve and function associated forming and consolidating memories which is why certain smells are so evocative of memory and emotion.

The olfactory nerve is actually a collection of nerve rootlets that extend down from the olfactory bulb (the branches that extend from the amygdala) and passed through the many openings within the cribriform plate located in the ethmoid bone. These specialized sensory receptive parts of the olfactory nerve are then located in the olfactory mucosa of the upper parts of the nasal cavity.   During breathing air molecules attach to the olfactory mucosa and stimulate the olfactory receptors of cranial nerve 1 and electrical activity is then transduced into the olfactory bulb. Olfactory bulb cells then transmit electrical activity to other parts of the central nervous system via the olfactory tract.

Issues Relating to the Olfactory Nerve

- Lesions to the olfactory nerve can occur because of blunt trauma, meningitis and tumors of the frontal lobe.

  Symptoms this nerve has been damaged: reduced ability to taste and smell. However, lesions of the olfactory nerve will not lead to a reduced ability to sense pain from the nasal epithelium. This is because pain from the nasal epithelium is not carried to the central nervous system by the olfactory nerve; rather, it is carried to the central nervous system by the trigeminal nerve (cranial nerve V). **Anosmia** is a lack of functioning olfaction, or an inability to perceive odors. Anosmia can be temporary or permanent. Causes could be due to birth trauma (if the function was never there) and genetics.

Smell disorders can have many causes. Most people who develop a smell disorder have recently experienced an illness (colds, upper respiratory infection) or a head injury. Other causes of smell disorders could be polyps in the nasal cavities, hormonal disturbances or dental problems. Exposure to chemicals, such as insecticides and solvents, and some medications have also been associated with smell disorders. People with head and neck cancers who receive radiation treatment are also among those who may experience problems with their sense of smell.

Sometimes, having a smell disorders can have serious consequences. The sense of smell often serves as a first warning signal, alerting us to the smoke of a fire or the odor of a natural gas leak and dangerous fumes. Sometimes a smell disorder can signal the underlining of a serious health problem such as diabetes, hypertension, chronic malnourishment, obesity Parkinson's disease, Alzheimer's disease, multiple sclerosis, and Korsakoff's disorder (a neurological disorder associated with severe lack of B1 due to complications associated with malnourishment and chronic alcoholism).

Structures Relating to the Olfactory Nerve
- **Amygdala**
- **Lateral Ventricles**

- **Falx**
- **Ethmoid Bone**
- **Heart**
- **The whole nervous system**

To Work with an Issue Relating to the Olfactory Nerve

Work with the whole, the limbic system, the ethmoid. Just be with it if it presents, no matter where you are holding in the body.

Cranial Nerve 2
Optic Nerve

The optic nerve begins at the back of the eye ball in a place called the optic disc. It travels through the optic canal, a fossa located within the sphenoid bone where it enters the middle cranial fossa where the nerves join the optic nerve from the other eye to form the optic chaisma. The optic chaisma sits just anteriorly to the pituitary stalk. Within the chaisma the nerves split) half the nerves axons cross midline to join the other non-crossed axons from the other eye), to become the optic tract that passes through the hypothalamus (an organ located below the thalamus and is an important brain structure that links nervous system function to the endocrine function via the pituitary gland (the pituitary gland is the master glad that regulates <u>all</u> hormone production in the body) where they act to influence the circadian rhythmus. * *The Circadian rhythms is roughly the 24 hour cycle of biochemical, physiological, and behavior processes of living entities. These rhythms allow organisms to anticipate and prepare for precise and regular environmental changes (biological clock), daytime, night time,* seasons. *They are important rhythmus to determine sleep and feeding as well as patterns of core body temperature, brain wave activity, hormone production, cell regulation and other biological activities associated to the daily cycle.* The optic tract then passes through the thalamus (an organ with two thalami located in the very central part of the brain one on each side of the third ventricle, this organ helps organizes where to send sensory and motor signals to various parts of the brain) and turns into the optic radiation, until it reaches the visual cortex in the occipital lobe at the very back of the brain. This is where the visual center of the brain is located and it will ultimately interpret electrical signals produced by light stimulation of the retina via the optic nerve as visual images.

The optic nerve is ensheathed with all three meningeal layers (dura, arachnoid and pia). This dural/meningeal attachment with the optic nerve makes they eyes literally and extension of the entire brain. Considered to be a part of the central nervous system, the optic nerve is derived from an out pouching of the diecenephalon (the earliest brain structure formed: the forebrain) during embryological development.

Function of the optic nerve is to transmit visual information from the retina to the brain. The preprocessing takes place in the retina and the signals are taken to the brain by the optic nerve.

Issues relating to the *Optic Nerve* - Injury to the optic nerve can be a result of congenital or heritable problems such as:

*Optic Neuritis – inflammation of the optic nerve. Symptoms are usually unilateral (only effecting one side), with eye pain feeling worse with eye movement and partial or complete vision loss. Cases often times resolve spontaneously. Inflammation of the optic nerve causes loss of vision usually because of the swelling and destruction of the myelin sheath covering the optic nerve. The most common disease associated with this condition is Multiple Sclerosis, in which cases there maybe recurrences and is often the presenting manifestation in diagnosis of M.S.

Other causes include:

- Infectious disease (viral encephalitis (particularly in children)), sinusitis, meningitis, TB, syphilis, HIV.
- Tumor metastasis (from another organ spreading or pressing) to the optic nerve.
- Chemicals and drugs (lead, methanol, arsenic, antibiotics).
- Rare causes include diabetes, pernicious anemia, Graves' disease, bee stings, and Trauma.

*Papilledema – swelling of the optic disc due to increased intercranial pressure and is almost always bilateral. Vision is not affected initially, but seconds-long graying out, flickering, blurred or double vision may occur. Patients may have increased symptoms of increased intercranial pressure, such as headaches or nausea and vomiting. This condition requires an immediate search for the cause.

Some major causes include:

- Cerebral trauma or hemorrhage
- Brain tumor or abscess
- Meningitis

- Arachnoidal adhesion (inflammation in the arachnoid which can sometimes lead to scaring that can make the nerves stick together.
- Cavernous or dural sinus thrombosis (blood clot)
- Encephalitis (inflammation of the brain usually due to virus, bacteria, parasite or fungi)
- Indiopathic intercranial hypertension (a condition with elevated CSF pressure and no mass lesion).

*Toxic Ambyopia – Reduction in visual acuteness or perception as the result of a toxic reaction or malnutrition. The vision loss is typically bilateral, painless, and (unless under extreme toxic reaction) does not cause profound vision loss.

*Ischemic Optic Neuropathy - Tissue death of the optic disc. The only constant symptom is painless vision loss, typically rapid (over minutes, hours, or days). Most causes are unilateral with bilateral cases being more uncommon. The optic disc swelling with the surrounding hemorrhages. Treatment is ineffective. Some symptoms are general malaise (feeling out of sorts), muscle aches and pains, headache over temple, pain when combing hair, pain in the jaw when chewing, temple arteritis (inflammation of the blood vessels in the head). However, symptoms may not occur until after vision loss.

- Nonarteritic – 50yrs or older
- Arteritic – 70 yrs or older (tends not to be as severe).

*Hereditary Optic Neuropathies – Genetic defects that cause vision loss, occasionally with cardiac or neurological abnormalities. Typically manifests in childhood or adolescence with bilateral, symmetric (identical in each eye) vision loss. Optic nerve damage is usually permanent and in some cases progressive. By the time optic atrophy is detected, substantial nerve injury has already occurred.

- <u>Dominant Optic Atrophy</u> – Premature degeneration of the optic nerve leading to progressive vision loss. Onset the 1st decade of life.

- <u>Leber's Hereditary Optic Neuropathy</u> – Involves mitochondrial DNA abnormality that effects cellular respiration. Although the whole body is affected, vision loss is the primary manifestation. Males affected 80% -90% of the time. Only females can pass on this abnormality, because the zygote receives mitochondria only from the mother.

*Glaucoma – disease involving loss of retinal ganglion cells causing optic neuropathy in a pattern of peripheral vision loss, initially sparing central vision. When left untreated it can lead to permanent damage to the optic nerve and progressive vision loss that can lead to blindness.

*Trauma, Infection (very rare), Compression from Tumors, Aneurysms

* Damage *before* the optic chiasm causes loss of vision on the same side as the damage.

* Damage *in* the chiasm causes loss of vision bilaterally.

* Damage *after* the chiasm causes loss of vision on the opposite side of the lesion but can affect both visual fields.

Structures Relating to the Optic Nerve
The structures relating to the optic nerve would be the sphenoid, the menigeal layers of the cranial vault, thalamus, hypothalamus, occipital lobe (occiput).

To Work with an Issue Associated with the Optic Nerve
- Could work with the:
- Sphenoid
- Sphenoibasilar Junction
- Occiput
- RTM – tentorium (vault hold) b/c this structure is so close anatomically to the optic nerve and connected fascially to the same menigeal layers.
- Lateral Ventricle
- Upper Thoracic
- Cervicals
- For inflammation I could hold the eyes if the client felt safe with that.
- Feet when working with blindness to ground and support the person low in the body, especially if the loss of vision was recent.

Cranial Nerve 3
Oculomotor Nerve

There are two nuclei for the oculomotor nerve:

- *The Oculomotor Nuclei- motor portion*

- *The Edingar-Westphal Nuclei*

Both nuclei originate in the *Superior Colliculus* of the *Mesencephalon (Midbrain)*

The *Superior Colliculus* (SC) is a major component of all vertebrate species. The general system of the SC is to direct behavior responses toward specific points in the ego centric (body-centered) space. In other words, it receives input from the eyes, produces gaze shifts, also accompanying the head and neck movement in orientation to the gaze. It is found that the SC is not needed for object recognition but plays a critical role in the ability to direct behaviors toward specific objects and can support this ability to direct even in the absence of the cerebral cortex. Overall, the SC encodes the target of gaze shifts calling movement to head and neck when needed, but does not seem to specify the precise movements needed to get there.

The nerve emerges from the SC at the interpeduncular fossa on the ventricle aspect of the mid-brain. * *The interpeduncular fossa – a deep depression on the inferior surface of the mesencephalon (mid-brain) between the two cerebral peduncles.* It then passes between the posterior and superior cerecellar arteries the nerve travels anteriorly into the cavernous sinus by piercing the dura anterior and lateral to the posterior clnoid processes of the sphenoid, passing between the free and attached borders of the Tentorium, and enters the cavernous sinus here, where it runs along the lateral wall of the sinus (also lateral to the internal carotoid artery) above the other orbital nerves. It continues forward through the superior orbital fissure to enter the orbit at the tendinous ring where it splits into superior and inferior branches. The superior branch innervates the superior rectus and the levator palpebrea muscles of the eye. While the inferior branch innervates the medial rectus, inferior rectus and inferior oblique muscles. The rest of the nerve bundles into the ciliary ganglion (a ganglion is an energy center/bundle) where it sees constriction of the iris (pupil) and the circular fibers of the ciliary muscles (accommodates vision). Basically, this nerve innervates all of the six muscles (this group of muscles are called the extraocular muscles) that control movement of the eyes except for one (the superior oblique muscle is innervated by the trochlear nerve).

Function of the oculomotor nucleus is to control *upward, downward, and adduction gaze* movement of the eye. And the function of the Edinger-Westphal nucleus is to the *ciliary ganglion* and *control pupil* *constriction* and ciliary muscle *vision accommodation* which is the apparatus of the eye that helps focus on a near object.

Issues Relating to the Oculomotor Nerve

*Ophthalmoparesis refers to paralysis of one or more of the extraocular muscles which are responsible for eye movement.

Causes can be the result from disorders of various parts of the eye and nervous system:

*Third Cranial (Oculomotor Nerve) Palsy – The effected eye turns outward while the unaffected eye look straight ahead causing double vision. The affected eye can only move to the middle when looking inward and cannot move up or down. Because the cranial nerve also raises the eye lid, the eye lid droops, and the pupil may be dilated. It may not constrict in response to light.

The underlining cause must be determined, especially if it has suddenly or gradually come on over time, for it could result in a very serious or life threatening condition.

Causes Include:

- Head Injury
- Aneurysm- a bulge in an artery supplying the brain
- Hemorrhage- bleeding
- Tumor

- Diabetes- A common occurrence, due to ischemic injury (a restriction of blood supply,) with type 3 diabetes of which the palsy tends to resolve itself over a period of months.
- Meningitis- is inflammation of the protective membranes covering the brain and spinal cord. There are some long term consequences of this illness including deafness, epilepsy, hydrocephalus (abnormal production of CSF in the brain), cognitive abnormalities, and oculomotor palsy.
- Demyelinating disease – like multiple sclerosis
- Microvascular diseases – a process in which small branches of arteries become damaged, like diabetes and auto-immune diseases (Graves's disease, Huntington's disease, etc)

Structures Relating to the Oculomotor Nerve

The structures relating to the oculomotor nerve would be the Superior Colliculus of the midbrain, the Interpeduncular fossa, and sphenoid, base of the tentorium, cavernous sinus, common tendinous ring, and the extraocular muscles.

To Work with an Issue Associated with the Oculomotor Nerve

Could work with:

- Holding the whole of the oculomotor nerve, pathway, and structures of the brain it connects to at the occiput.

- Hold specifically the Interpeduncular fossa which is situated directly in the middle of the brain and where the nerve emerges from the mesencephalon.

- Cavernous sinus

- Tentorium

- Temporals

- Sutherland's fulcrum

- Eyes even if it felt resourcing to the client to be held there and they were requesting that kind of contact.

- Sphenoid

- SBJ

- Cervicals and it relation to the midbrain

- Basically in Biodynamics we could hold the structures of the oculomotor nerve from just about anywhere in the body. As long as we are holding the whole and inquiring about what is softer, slower, longer, more fluid, less compressed, etc while resonating within our own body tissue to fluid filling, softness, and being neutral in our seat.

Cranial Nerve 4
Trochlear Nerve

The *Trochlear Nerve* is a motor nerve (somatic efferent) that innervates a single muscle (*Superior Oblique Muscle*) of the eye.

Unique among the nerve:

*It is the smallest nerve in terms of the number of axons it contains.

*It has the greatest intracranial length.

*Along with the optic nerve, it is the only cranial nerve that decussates (crosses to the other side) before innervating its target.

*It is the only cranial nerve that exists from the dorsal aspect of the brainstem.

The nucleus of the 4th (trochlear) nerve is located in the *Tegmentum of the mid brain* at the level of the *Inferior Colliculus* just caudal (nearer the tail of the body) to the lateral nucleus of the 3rd (oculomotor) nerve.

The *Midbrain Tegmentum* controls motor function, regulates awareness and attention, and is involved in an assortment of autonomic functions that have to do with homeostasis and reflex.

The *Inferior Colliculus* has relation to the auditory system.

The nerve emerges from the midbrain dorsally coming from around the *Periaqueductal Gray* Matter surrounding the *cerebral aqueduct* (a fluid filled space of CSF connecting the 3rd ventricle, in the Diencephalon, to the 4th ventricle, between the Pons and Cerebellum). It then crosses midline at this dorsal or posterior aspect of the midbrain, just caudally to the *Inferior Colliculus*. Then travels in the subarachnoid space around the *Cerebral Peduncles* to pass the *Posterior and Superior Cerebellar Arteries*, just lateral to the 3rd cranial nerve (Oculomotor). It penetrates the dura behind and lateral to the *Posterior Clinoid Process* entering the *Cavernous Sinus* where it runs just inferior to CN3. The nerve enters the orbit through the *Superior Orbital Fissure* moving above the *Tendinous Ring*, to innervate the *Superior Oblique Muscle* of the eye.

Function: is to provide movement to the Superior Oblique Muscle. The allowable movement of this muscle is (1) looking up and down (2) and rotation in the plane of face with intorsion and extorsion of the eye ball.

Issues Relating to the Trochlear Nerve

Fourth Nerve (Trochlear Nerve) Palsy – The long course of the Trochlear nerve can make it susceptible to injury especially associated with head trauma. There are two types of manifestations of damage:

- Vertical Diplopia (double vision) – causes weakness of downward eye movement where the effected eye drifts upward relative to the normal eye. To compensate for this, the patient learns to tilt the head forward (tucking the chin in) in order to bring the field of vision back together. The diplopia gets worse when looking toward the nose.

- Torsional Diplopia – causes torsion (rotation of the eye ball in the plane of the face). Naturally, torsion is a normal response to tilting the head sideways, so that the orientation of the environment remains unchanged. The characteristic appearance is head tilt to one side, chin tucked in; however, other causes must be ruled out b/c torticollis (weakness in the neck) can produce a similar appearance.

The most common cause identified to this repercussion is head injury. Occasionally, diabetes can cause this type of palsy. Rarely, the cause of a tumor, an aneurysm, or multiple sclerosis is to blame but it does happen. In these causes the injury can get better or heal over time with the right treatment. Sometimes they call for surgery. A chronic case is most often due to birth defects and maybe noticed at birth or childhood with major defects. However, minor cases may not become evident until adulthood.

Structures Relating to the Trochlear Nerve

The structure relating to the Trochlear nerve would be Inferior Colliculus of the Midbrain, Cerebral Aqueduct, and the Subarachnoid Space around the Cerebral Peduncles, Superior and Posterior Cerebellar Arteries, Tentorium, Cavernous Sinus, Internal Carotid Artery, Superior Orbital Fissure of the Sphenoid, Superior Oblique Muscle.

To Work with an Issue Associated with the Trochlear Nerve

Sphenoid
Holding at the occiput to support the nucleus of the nerve and facilitating nourishment to the cerebral aqueduct.

Hold the Temporals to support softening of the tentorium where the nerve pierces the dura there.

Could work with the Cervicals to decompress tension in the midbrain.

Hold with the intention of supporting the nerve and the whole system and ask where it wants to be supported.

Hold Sutherland Fulcrum of which the nerve sits in front.

Hold the blood in the arteries it articulates with.

Listening always.

Cranial Nerve 5
Trigeminal Nerve

This nerve is the largest cranial nerve. And the nerve is also one of the first cranial nerves to develop in utero which is nearly completely form by 2 months.

The Tri in Trigeminal Nerve means three. **This nerve has 3 major branches**:

- Ophthalmic division (V1)

- Maxillary division (V2)

- Mandibular division (V3)

It has both sensory and motor roots of function:

Its <u>sensory root</u> is responsible for most of the sensations in the face, while its <u>motor root</u> innervate the muscles of mastication or chewing.

The Trigeminal Nerve has 4 nuclei in the brain stem which 3 of them are sensory. All together they extends down from the Pons of the midbrain into the spinal cord all the way to about C2 or C3. This nucleus is composed of *3 sub nuclei*:

- *Mesencephalic* nucleus = receives *proprioceptive information* for the muscles of *mastication* which is the *projected* to the motor nucleus to provide reflex control of bite.

- *Pontine* Trigeminal nucleus or *Main* Sensory nucleus = concerned primarily with discriminative sense and *touch sensations for the face, nasal, and oral cavities.*

- *Spinal* nucleus = receiving perception of *Pain* and *Temperature.*

Both the large sensory root and the small motor root *emerge* from the brainstem at the *mid-lateral* surface of the *Pons*.

The 3 branches converge in the *trigeminal (Gasserian) ganglion* located within *Meckel's Cave*, and contain cell bodies of the incoming sensory nerve fibers.

Meckel's Cave – *is situated in a cavern within the middle cranial fossa of the sphenoid. The "cave" consists of:*

 *Tentorium (supero-laterally)

 *Lateral wall of the Cavernous Sinus (supero-medially)

 *Clivus (medially)

 *Posterior Petrous Face (infero-laterally)

The nerve then branches off into:

The Ophthalmic nerve which carries the sensory information from the scalp and forehead, upper eyelid, conjunctiva (thin covering of the whites in the eye) and cornea (thin covering of the iris and pupil) of the eye , the upper and tip of the nose, the nasal mucosa, frontal sinuses, and parts of the dura and blood vessels there (meninges)

The Maxillary nerve carries the sensory information from the lower eyelid and cheeks, the nares (openings of the nose) and the upper lip, the upper teeth and gums, the nasal mucosa, palate and the roof of the pharynx, maxillary, ethmoid and sphenoid sinuses, and parts of the meninges.

The Mandibular nerve carries the sensory information from the lower lip, teeth, gums, chin, jaw, parts of the external ear, and parts of the meninges. The Mandibular nerve also has a motor pathway which is responsible for movement involved in biting, chewing, and swallowing. It innervates also the masseter, temporalis, medial and lateral pterygoids, tensor veli palatine, myohyoid, anterior belly of digastrics, and tensor tympani muscles.

Issues Relating to the Trigeminal Nerve

- **Trigeminal Neuralgia** – is facial nerve pain sometimes accompanied with a brief facial spasm or tic. The symptoms are sudden unilateral, severe, brief, stabbing, sharp, and sometimes like electric shocks, lasting for a few seconds to a few minutes. Some triggers include being touched in certain places on the face, eating, and shaving, applying makeup, brushing teeth, smiling, drinking, encountering a breeze, and talking. The symptoms have to potential to come and go, while also going into remission at times. This condition is one of the most common causes of facial pain, although the condition itself is rare.

Causes include:

Pressure of a blood vessel on the root of the trigeminal nerve.

Demyelinization of the nerve, also appearing in advanced stages of MS.

Pressure of a tumor on the trigeminal nerve (rare)

Physical damage to the nerve caused by dental or surgical procedures, injury to the face or infections.

Unknown cases.

Can occur in all nerve disorders.

Shingles

Head trauma

There can be other problems associated with this nerve:

Problems with the sensory parts result in pain or loss of sensations in the face. Problems with the motor root result in deviation of the jaw toward the affected side and trouble chewing.

Structure Relating to the Trigeminal Nerve

The structures relating to the trigeminal nerve would be around C1, C2, and possibly C3,

Pons, sphenoid, base of the reciprocal tension membrane, Meckel's Cave, mandible, maxilla, ethmoid, frontal bone, nose.

To Work with an Issue Associated with the Trigeminal Nerve

Holding the whole
Sphenoid
Occiput

Cervicals

Frontal Bone

Maxilla

Mandible (Jaw)

Vault Hold

Work with finding resources in the body

Anywhere along the spinal cord

Cranial Nerve 6
Abducens Nerve

Function: To control one single muscle in the eye; to contract the Lateral Rectus Muscle resulting in abduction of the eye.

The nucleus is located in the ventrical aspect of the *Pons, just to the floor of the Fourth Ventricle, close to midline* (like the other nuclei that control eye movement; Oculomotor and the Trochlear).

The nerve cells *exit* the brain stem *at* the site where the *Pons* comes into junction with the *Pyramid of Medulla*. From there they travel anteriorly where it pierces the *Dura* lateral to the *Dorsum Sellae of the Sphenoid*. The nerve continues forward and bends over the ridge of the *Petrous on the Temporalis Bone*, where it then enters the *Cavernous Sinus*. It passes lateral to the *Carotid Artery* before it enters the *Superior Orbital Fissure*, passing also through the

Tendinous Ring to enter the deep surface of the *Lateral Rectus Muscle.*

Issues Relating to the Abducens Nerve

Peripheral Lesions – complete interruption of the sixth (Abducens) nerve can cause diplopia (double vision). In order for patients to see without the double vision, they will rotate their heads so both eyes are looking sideways.

Causes

Tumors, aneurysms, fracture, or basically anything that directly compresses or stretched the nerve. Other processes that can disrupt the vision in this way include stroke, demyelination, infections like meningitis, cavernous sinus disease and other neuropathies, diabetic Neuropathy (which is one of the leading causes., Wernicke – Korsakoff syndrome Caused by thiamine deficiency classically due to alcoholism, and Tolosa-Hunt syndrome.

Nuclear Lesions – damage to the nucleus creates a horizontal gaze palsy (the eye gets stuck) that affects both eyes simultaneously.

Supranuclear Lesions – involves conjugate gaze, not unilateral eye movement.

Structures Relating to the Abducens Nerve

The structures relating to the abducens nerve would be the Midbrain (specifically where the Pons and pyramid of the Medulla junction) , Fourth ventricle, Midline, Sphenoid, base of the RTM, Cavernous sinus, Superior Orbital Fissure of the sphenoid, Temporal Bone, Tendinous Ring, Lateral Rectus Muscle.

To Work with an Issue of the Abducens Nerve

Could work with:
Holding the whole of the Abducens Nerve, pathway, and structures of the brain it is in contact with while working anywhere on the body.
Sphenoid
Temporals
RTM
Midbrain
Venous Sinuses

Cranial Nerve 7
Facial Nerve

Emerging from the brainstem between the Pons and the Medulla; the *motor root* sits in the *facial nerve nucleus* in the Pons, while the *sensory root* sits in the *nervus intermedius* which also host its parasympathetic fibers. A dural sleeve covers the motor and sensory roots of the facial nerve. The nerve pierces the dura at the fundus of the internal acoustic meatus. From here the nerve has a rather complicated course through the brain:

The motor aspect of the nerve moves away from the midbrain and enters a canal of the *Petrous of the Temporal Bone*. Here is where it enters the inner ear at the *Internal Auditory Meatus* (or Internal Acoustic Meatus) along with other hearing and balance nerves.

The nerve then runs a very long a twisty path through the *Facial Canal* (the longest osseous (bone) canal of a nerve in humans) where it enters the middle ear compartment wrapping around the smallest of three bones behind the eardrum before emerging from the *Styomastoid Foramen of the Temporal Bone* (between the styloid and mastoid processes).

Upon exiting the Stylomastoid Foramen it travels outside of the skull to *pass through the Parotid Gland* where it then *divides* into five major branches to make multiple places of *contact* with facial muscles. (Although, it passes through the parotid gland it does not innervate the gland. The nerve that is responsible for that innervation is the glossopharyngeal cranial nerve). The Parotid gland is the largest of the salivary glands and sits behind the tongue in the back of the throat.

The Parasympathetic aspect of the nerve supplies ganglions of the parasympathetic nervous system on the head and neck making this nerve connected to the Ventral aspect of the Vagus Nerve which is tied to our Social Engagement Nervous System. The engagement of the vagus nerve helps to regulate eye gaze, facial expressions, the ability to listen, and the use of rhythm and tone in our voices to convey emotions. In turn, this specific aspect of the nervous system can be used to calm the heart beat, generate digestive abilities, and calm the nervous system overall including both aspects (sympathetic and parasympathetic).

In Embryology, this nerve is developmentally derived from the Hyoid arch.

Function: This nerve is responsible for muscle control of the face. Hence, controls most facial expressions, secretion of tears and saliva, taste from the front part of the tongue.

Voluntary facial movements, such as wrinkling the brow, showing teeth, frowning, closing the eyes tightly, pursing the lips and puffing out the cheeks, all test the facial nerve. There should be no noticeable asymmetry.

Issues Relating to the Facial Nerve

Nervus Intermedius (Geniculate Neralgia) – A Severe stabbing pain centered directly and deep in the ear. Possibly, beginning gradually, becoming dull, possibly persistent, and sharp or stabbing, like electric shock, deep in the ear. It is a disorder associated with damage or inflammation to the nucleus of the 7th facial nerve. The pain can be triggered by swallowing or talking with possible pain free periods in between. Rarely do patients have pain in the nervus intermedius territory. Sometimes accompanies with loss of taste, paralysis, and a decrease in salvation. It sometimes follows herpes zoster infection. Can be treated with medication.

Bell's Palsy - is a fairly common facial paralysis that can happen to this nerve. Usually only effecting one side of the face, its cause is due to damage to this nerve most common to disease in the internal auditory meatus that affects the actual nerve tract. It usually strikes over night and can be very frightening to the patient who wakes up and is unable to move one side of their face. Prognosis is for recovery over several months, and often recovery is complete.

Sometimes this condition can happen as the result of Lyme's Disease.

Idiopathic Disease – A condition that arises "mysteriously" and the medical community cannot determine a cause.

Physical Trauma to the Head particularly fractures of the Temporal bones can cause paralysis to this nerve.

Tumor

Herpes Zoster Oticus – patients present with facial paralysis. Ear pain, hearing loss, vertigo, and vacuoles.

Moebius Syndrome – this condition is a bilateral facial paralysis resulting from underdevelopment of the facial nerve which is present at birth and affects both the facial and abducens cranial nerves. The cause is widely unknown. However, there has been some thought that temporary loss of blood flow during the prenatal period maybe a result, either due to some kind of trauma in utero, drug use, etc.

Acute and Chronic Otitis Media (infection of the middle ear) can spread to the facial nerve and inflame it. Symptoms present with chronic discharge of the ear, or hearing loss, with or without ear pain. Medical attention is very important.

Structures Relating to the Facial Nerve

The structures relating to the facial nerve would be the Temporal Bones, Maxilla, Midbrain, Inner and Middle Ear, Facial Canal, RTM, Midbrain at the Pons, Vagus Nerve

To Work with an Issue Associated with the Facial Nerve

Could work with:

Vagus Nerve or the Sympathetic Ganglia Chain

Temporal Bones

RTM (tentorium at the base of the head)

Occiput (to hold the midbrain and the pons)

Maxilla

Vault Hold

Could work with the cranial bones that the branches travel too... Frontal Bone, Zygomatic arch, etc

Ears

Cranial Nerve 8
Vestibulocochlear Nerve

This nerve is <u>purely a sensory</u> nerve and its <u>Function:</u> is to transmit sound and equilibrium (balance/proprioception) information from the inner ear to the brain.

It contains <u>two nuclei</u> the *Vestibular Nucleus* and the *Cochlear Nucleus*.

Vestibular aspect of this cranial nerve has 4 subnuclei that are situated at the floor of the four ventricle.

- Medial Vestibular Nucleus

- Lateral Vestibular Nucleus

- Inferior Vestibular Nucleus

- Superior Vestibular Nucleus

This division on the Vestibulochlear Nerve *carries spatial orientation information from the semicircular canals*. The semicircular canals are three half-circular, interconnected tubes locates inside each ear, aligned roughly at a 45 degree angle to the vertical plane drawn from the nose to the back of the skull. Each canal is filled with fluid and contain motion sensor that are little hairs called cilia. As the head turns the fluid is thrown into different directions and the cilia detect when the fluid rushes past and sends a signal to the brain.

The cochlear aspect of this cranial nerve *carries the signals from the cochlea (auditory portion of the inner ear)* to the brain. There are 2 major components of the cochlear nuclear complex:

- Dorsal Cochlear Nucleus

- Ventral Cochlear Nucleus – further divided in to 2 components – anteroventral and posteroventral cochlear nucleus

The cochlea is filled with a watery liquid, which moves in response to the vibrations coming from the middle ear via the oval window. As the fluid moves, thousands of "hair cells" are set in motion, and convert that motion to electrical signals that are communicated via neurotransmitters to many thousands of nerve cells. These primary auditory neurons transform the signals into electrical impulses known as action potentials, which travel along the auditory nerve to structures in the brainstem for further processing.

The veribulocochlear nerve travels through the *internal auditory meatus in company* with the 7th cranial nerve, and enters the canal of the *Petrous of the Temporal Bone* also with the 7th (Facial) cranial nerve where it penetrates the brain stem in the area of the medulla at its junction with the pons at the base on the 4th ventrical. The *vestibular nerve aspect* terminates at the floor of the four ventrical. The axons of the *Cochlear Axons continues on to terminate* in the *Transverse Temporal Gyri* (also called *Heschl's Gyri*), founded in the *Primary Auditory Cortex* in the *Superior Temporal Gyrus* of the brain occupying *area 41.*

Issues Relating to the Vestibulocochlear Nerve

Damage to the vestibulochlear nerve may cause the following symptoms:

- **Hearing loss** – can be due to infection, heredity, meningitis, trauma, certain medications, long term exposure to loud noise, aging.

- **Vertigo**

- **False sense of motion**

- **Loss of equilibrium** (in dark places)

- **Motion sickness**

- **Nystagmus** - involuntary eye movement or unintentional jittery movement of the eyes associated, in the case involving the 8th cranial nerve, with proprioception being off balance.

- **Gaze-Evoked Tinnitus** - sudden loud ringing in ears with eye movement. (Very Rare)

- **Vestibulocochlear nerve disease** - involves lesions that form along the nerve which cause impaired hearing, vertigo, tinnitus, nausea, and balance problems.

- Sometimes **lesions on the Facial Nerve** can effect and put pressure on the vestiblocochlear nerve.

Structures Related to the Vestibulocochlear Nerve

The structures relating to the optic nerve would be the temporal bones, fourth ventricle, the menigeal layers especially area of the Tentorium cerebelli, Superior Temporal Gyrus, Internal Auditory Meatus

To Work with Issues Associated with the Vestibulocochlear Nerve

Work with the whole

Temporals

Illiac Crests or the sides of the pelvic bowl

Shoulder

Lungs

Work to settle the system as a whole working to slow things down (there is a lot of strain involved in the person who is struggling the hear).

Occiput

Feet

Glossopharyngeal Nerve
Cranial Nerve 9

This nerve relates to the tongue and the pharynx.

Function – Swallowing, Gag Reflex, and Speech

Sensory Function:

- This nerve receives general sensory fibers along the ventral trigeminothalamic tract which entails the tonsils, pharynx, the middle ear, and the posterior 1/3 of the tongue. (The Ventral Trigeminlthalamic Tract serves as pain, temperature, and light touch pathway from the face, head and neck. It receives input from 4 cranial nerves total: The Trigeminal, Facial, Glossopharyngeal, and Vagus nerves).

- The area that innervates the posterior part of the tongue has special nerve fibers that enable the sensation of taste.

- It also receives visceral sensory information from the carotid bodies which are little clusters of cell bodies that detect changes in the composition of arterial blood flowing through it, mainly the partial of oxygen, but also carbon dioxide, and it is also sensitive to changes in pH and temperature which are located along the carotid artery.

- It also supplies parasympathetic fibers to the <u>parotid gland</u> the largest of the salvitory glands:

via the <u>optic ganglion:</u>

- The Glossopharyngeal nerve also contributes to the parasympathetic sensory mechanism of the <u>Pharyngeal Plexus</u> which consists of a network of nerve fibers innervating most of the palate, larynx, and pharynx. (Along with the vagus nerve)

Motor Function – This nerve sole motor function supplies the motor ability of the <u>stylopharyngeus muscle</u>.

Pathway:

The nucleus of the Glossopharyngeal nerve resides between the Olivary body (sometimes called the olive and *marks the swollen region between the anterolateral and posterolateral sulci in the upper part of the medulla. The mass is caused by gray matter known as the inferior olivary nucleus: which is associated with the cerebellum, meaning that it is involved in control and coordination of movements*) and the inferior cerebellar peduncle of the medulla oblongata (the lower part of the brain stem).

The nerve immediately exits *the skull through the Jugular Foramen* in its own sheath of dura mater just lateral and anterior to the vagus and accessory nerve, between the internal jugular vein and the internal carotid artery, beneath the styloid process and the muscles connected to it, to lay upon the styopharyngeus and middle pharungeal constrictor muscle, traveling to pass under cover of the hyoplossus muscle to finally distribute to the palatine tonsil, the mucus membrane of the fauces and the base of the tongue, and the mucous glands of the mouth.

The Glossopharyngeal Nerve Branches:

- Tympanic – branch found near the ear

- Stylopharygeal – a muscle of the neck

- Tonsillar – innervates the tonsils

- Nerve to carotid sinus – communicates with the Vagus Nerve here and the sympathetic nervous system through the carotid body to help maintain consistent blood pressure.

- Branches to the posterior third of tongue – taste and sensation

Issues Relating to the Glossopharyngeal Nerve

- **Glossopharyngeal Neuralgia** – Consists of recurring attacks of severe pain in the back of the throat, the area near the tonsils, the back of the tongue, and part of the ear. The pain is due to malfunction of the 9th cranial nerve (glossopharyngeal nerve), which moves the muscles of the throat and carries information from the throat, tonsils, and tongue to the brain. This disorder is rare and not very widely understood.

Some cause include:

- Abnormal positioned artery that compresses the glossopharyngeal nerve.

- Compression at the Jugular Foreman due to head injury.

- The case of a tumor in the brain or neck (rarely).

Symptoms: Excruciating painful attacks possibly triggered by a particular action such as chewing, swallowing, talking, coughing, or sneezing. The pain usually begins at the back of the tongue or back of the throat, while sometimes spreading to the ear, lasting several seconds to a few minutes. It most commonly effects only one side. In 1 to 2% of people who experience this may have their heart beat affected, where it slows the heart lowering blood pressure, even to the point where the heart could stop temporarily, causing fainting. This mechanism for the fall in blood pressure and heart rate is not well understood; however, it must disturb the carotid bodies and their function and communication to the vagus nerve.

Allopathic Treatment: Medication and /or Surgery. It is diagnosis is determined if a local anesthetic eliminates the pain. MRI should be done to check for tumors.

Structures Relating to the Glossopharyngeal Nerve

Temporal Bone
Medulla Oblongata
Vagus Nerve

Accessory Nerve
Occiput Bone
The Fourth Ventricle
Base of the Tentorium
All the muscles attached to the styloid process
The Heart

To Work with an Issue Associated with the Glossopharyngeal Nerve
Work with the whole while inquiring about what is deeper then the
issue at hand, softer, wider, longer, while being neutral in our seat.

Cranial Nerve 10
Vagus Nerve

Vagus is Latin for "wandering". This merges at the back of the skull
and meanders in a leisurely way through the abdomen, with a
number of branching nerves coming into contact with the heart,
lungs, voicebox, stomach, and ears, among other body parts. The
vagus nerve carries incoming information from the nervous system
to the brain, providing information about what the body is doing,
and it also transmits outgoing information which governs a range of
reflex responses associated with the parasympathetic nervous
system. **The Vagus Nerve is one of the many vital nerves that keep
your body in working order. It is the main nerve associated with the
Parasympathetic Nervous System.** The vagus nerve helps to regulate
the heart beat, controls muscle movement, keep a person breathing,
helps to transmit a variety of chemicals through the body. It is also

responsible for keeping the digestive tract in working order, contracting the muscles of the stomach and intestines to help process food, and sending back information about what is being digested and what the body is getting out of it.

Pathway

The Vagal fibers are connected to four nuclei in the Medulla (Brainstem) which then translate into the four branches of the nerve after it exits the cranial vault via the jugular foramen (see pictures below):

- **The Spinal Nucleus of the Trigeminal Nerve *(general sensory)*** – carries sensations (*pain, touch, temperature, vibration, and proprioceptive*) from the posterior meninges, concha, skin at the back of the ear and the external acoustic meatus, part of the external surface of the tympanic membrane, the pharynx, and larynx. (<u>This nuclei is basically dealing with these aspects of the facial nerve</u>).

- **The Nucleus of the Tractus Solitaries *(visceral sensory)*** – *carries visceral sensations* ('feel good' or 'feel bad' body sensations; or perceives sensory input ,except pain, from the viscera) from the larynx, trachea on the caudal part, esophagus, and all the thoracic and abdominal viscera, stretch receptors in the wall of the aortic arch, and the chemoreceptors in the aortic bodies adjacent to the arch.

- **The Nucleus Ambiguous *(branchial motor)*** – *carries out motor ability* to the superior, middle, and inferior constrictors, levator palate, salpingopharyngeus, and one muscle of the tongue, the palatoglossus, via the pharyngeal plexus and to cricothyroid and intrinsic muscles of the larynx.

- **The Dorsal Vagal Motor Nucleus** *(parasympathetic visceral motor)* -   innervates the viscera, including glands and all smooth muscle of the pharynx, larynx, all thoracic and abdominal viscera: Cardiac Muscles.

The Vagus nerve fibers emerges from their nuclei within the medulla of the brain stem dorsal to the olive as 8 or 10 rootlets caudal to those of the glossopharyngeal nerve (CN9).

These rootlets converge into a flat cord that exits the skull through the jugular foramen.

There are two sensory ganglia associated with the vagus nerve. They are the superior and inferior vagal ganglia which are located directly either within or immediately following the exit out of the jugular foramen. (*Ganglia are dense group of nerve cell bodies present in most animals that carry impulses throughout the body)*

After passing through the Jugular Foramen and the Ganglia, the nerve branches out to wonder through the organs of the neck, thorax, and abdomen.

Branches of the Vagus Nerve

- **Auricular nerve**
- **Pharyngeal nerve**
- **Superior laryngeal nerve**
- **Superior cervical cardiac branches of vagus nerve**
- **Inferior cervical cardiac branch**
- **Recurrent laryngeal nerve**
- **Thoracic cardiac branches**
- **Branches to the pulmonary plexus**
- **Branches to the esophageal plexus**
- **Anterior vagal trunk**
- **Posterior vagal trunk**

Parasympathetic innervation of the heart is mediated by the vagus nerve. Specifically, the vagus nerve acts to lower the heart rate.

Issues Relating to the Vagus Nerve

Activation of the vagus nerve typically leads to a reduction in heart rate, blood pressure, or both. Excessive activation of the vagal nerve during emotional stress, which is a parasympathetic overcompensation of a strong sympathetic nervous system response associated with stress, can also cause vasovagal syncope because of a sudden drop in blood pressure and heart rate. Vasovagal syncope affects young children and women more often. It can also lead to temporary loss of bladder control under moments of extreme fear.

- **Fainting - *Vagus Nerve Stimulation:*** Fainting may occur if the vagus nerve, which supplies the neck, chest, and intestine, is stimulated. When stimulated, the vagus nerve slows the heart. Such stimulation also causes nausea and cool, clammy skin. This type of fainting is called vasovagal (vasomotor) syncope. The vagus nerve is stimulated by pain, fear, other distress (such as that due to the sight of blood), vomiting, a large bowel movement, and urination. Fainting during or immediately after urination is called Micturition or Vasovagal syncope. Rarely, vigorous swallowing causes fainting due to stimulation of the vagus nerve.

- **Hiatal Hernias maybe caused by/ or create a pinching of the Vagus Nerve -** In a Hiatus Hernia, or Hiatal Hernia, the upper portion of the stomach protrudes through the opening (hiatus) in the diaphragm muscle. This condition may also manifest allergy like symptoms to food as well as cause reflux irritations throughout the body. \

- **Surgery –** Especially in the Abdominal cavity has been known to cause Vagus nerve damage, either due to cutting the nerve or scar tissue restricting the nerve. Symptoms include all kind of irritable bowel syndrome like constipation, trouble eliminating, acid reflux, gag reflex and swallowing problems.

- **Gastroparesis -** also called delayed gastric emptying, is a disorder in which the stomach takes too long to empty its contents. Normally, the stomach contracts to move food down into the small intestine for digestion. The vagus nerve controls the movement of food from the stomach through the digestive tract. Gastroparesis occurs when the vagus nerve is damaged and the muscles of the stomach and intestines do not work normally. Food then moves slowly or stops moving through the digestive tract.

Causes - The most common cause of gastroparesis is diabetes. People with diabetes have high blood glucose, also called blood sugar, which in turn causes chemical changes in nerves and damages the blood vessels that carry oxygen and nutrients to the nerves. Over time, high blood glucose can damage the vagus nerve. Some other causes of gastroparesis are

- surgery on the stomach or vagus nerve
- viral infections
- anorexia nervosa or bulimia
- medications—anticholinergics and narcotics—that slow contractions in the intestine
- gastroesophageal reflux disease
- smooth muscle disorders, such as amyloidosis and scleroderma
- nervous system diseases, including abdominal migraine and Parkinson's disease
- metabolic disorders, including hypothyroidism

Many people have what is called idiopathic gastroparesis, meaning the cause is unknown and cannot be found even after medical tests.

- In relation to Autoimmune disorders it was discovered in 2007 that the 'vagus nerve speaks directly to the immune system through a neurochemical called acetylcholine. And stimulating the vagus nerve sent commands to the immune system to stop pumping out toxic inflammatory markers.' New research in vagus stimulation is being conducted at a way to treat active auto immune disorders. Thus, working with the vagus nerve with patients suffering from 'active' autoimmune disorders could prove useful.

- Working with the vagus nerve can be beneficial for people dealing with Epilepsy and Low Blood Pressure.

- Diseases of the tenth cranial nerve, including **brain stem lesions** involving its nuclei (solitary, ambiguus, and dorsal motor), nerve fascicles, and intracranial and extracranial course. Clinical manifestations may include dysphagia, vocal cord weakness, and alterations of parasympathetic tone in the thorax and abdomen.

- Any kind of spasm in the abdominal or thoracic region could be caused by the vagus nerve.

- Whiplash could cause much dysfunction in this nerve, the parasympathetic nervous system while over producing stimulation of the sympathetic nervous system and also causing problems for the accessory nerve.

Structure Relating to the Vagus Nerve

- **Temporal bones**
- **Sternocleidomastoid or any of the muscles in the neck**
- **Occiput**
- **All the organs within the abdominal and thoracic cavity**
- **Respiratory Diaphram**
- **Falx or Tentorium**
- **Clavicles**
- **Stomach**

- **TMJ**
- **Upper Ribs**
- **Iliopoas**
- **The Entire Digestive System**
- **The Parasympathetic Nervous System and the Sympathetic Nervous System as a whole**

To Work with an Issue Relating to the Vagus Nerve

Work anywhere and hold the whole. Hold an organ and hold the whole. Hold the CranioVault and hold the whole. What is softer, wider, longer, deeper, less restricted. Work with resources especially around a dysfunction around this nerve b/c there may be sympathetic nervous system over load happening.

Chapter Eleven

How to Work with Still Points

As a clinical application when you notice imbalance- We work to slow these rhythms down. When they come up fast the system is working out of the CRI. As practitioners we are always asking the body what is deeper, longer, slower, wider, smoother. It is from a settled, slower place that the body can readjust itself. Similar to how sleeping rejuvenates the body. Helping the body to slow down and possible come to still point can help the body release un-useful patterns. When a practitioner can see and feel how the patterns of motion relate to the whole it is like an acknowledgement to the clients system. By acknowledging the system the practitioner can encourage a still point (where the body's inherent health lives) and access to the deepest realms of health and healing in the physical body.

- **Listen**
- **Acknowledge the Pattern**
- **Ask how it relates to the whole**
- **What is Deeper, Longer, Wider, Smoother, Slower**
- **Practitioner resources their own system by encouraging stillness within their own system with presence and listening, knowing, thinking, seeing   hands floating like corks.**
- **Once stillness arises in the clients system stay present and support until you notice movement arising again. Once the movement arises again listen to see if the pattern has shifted or changed before moving to a different hold.**

Still point is where the potency is building or re-charging in the system. As long as the client feels resourced and at peace let them remain in still point until the movement arises again. Often times the system can feel like there is a sparkly essence deep inside or a bubbly feeling. Sometimes it just feels like a holy presence underneath the skin. If the tissues feel like no-body is home the person may be in shut down and you will want to check-in with them by asking what they are noticing in their body. If they are in true still point they may be in a dream like state like a journeying experience or feeling peaceful and quite. It they are in a shut down state they can be activated in a past memory of trauma or stuck in an uncomfortable way either emotionally or physically having pain or discomfort in some way.

Developing Presence Skills: Introduction to maintaining a wide perceptual field by tuning into self and the client from a quite centered place **(Practitioner Neutral)**

Role of the Practitioner

- Settling into mid-line.

- Thinking fluids full body.

- Using "thinking, seeing, knowing hands" floating like corks on top of water.

- Orientation in a field of resonating.

Note: If you lose track of where you are or what is happening now, if you leave the present moment and come into thinking/planning mind:

- *Come back to roots*
- *Come back to Breath*
- *Come back to mid-line*
- *Come back to the energetic quality of the heart*
- *Come back to feet*

And……

wait for the Breath of Life to reveal itself.
Learning to sense the rhythm:

- Listening at the feet, occiput, sacrum and respiratory diaphragm with a developing sense of Presence of the whole (Floating Hands that are Listening). *Go over Anatomy Slides for Occiput and Sacrum.* Relate how these bones are connected to the primitive streak and good listening points for fluid dynamics.

- Demonstrate self care for the therapist as they listen for rhythms

- Talk about using light touch 5 grams of pressure to feel these motions

The Role of Muscle Memory in the Craniosacral System

The Body always Remembers and the Body always Knows what it needs to be in Balance

- o *When clients come in for sessions, they come in with a number of different emotions, stories, and histories in the foreground.*

- o Conditions that tend to have emotional components:

- ▪ Chronic Pain Sites
- ▪ Organs
- ▪ Areas the body might be protecting

- New/Old Trauma Sites
  - As Craniosacral Therapist we work with the Blueprint which can be linked to the Primitive Streak that is laid down during the embryological development of the embryo before the rooting/nesting phase. The Blue Print is always present even in the face of grave traumas, injury, pain, illness and disease. This Blue Print is always resting deep inside and is very still. Anatomically, it rests within the circular vertebral bodies of the spine (site where remnant cells of the photonic primitive streak exist). This Blue Print embodies the inherent Health of all beings. For it was the essence of our original intention before our histories and is our birth-rite to be able to live in harmony with this physiological remembrance (refer to Jaap van der Wal).

  - The PRI is all the physiological parts that move the CSF which posses an electric sparkly phosphorescence that is not present when we die. As Craniosacral Therapist we come to support the health that is already there and trust the Breath of Life and the Tides to organize more and more deeply around the Blue Print. We do this by being **Still**, **Listening** with our hands, being **Present** in out body, sustaining a practitioner **Neutral** that is non-judging and free of an agenda for the client. We also hold this Health by understanding that the Body and all the forces that hold us to our stories, or pain, our injuries, our illnesses are operating out of the highest organization of Balance and Heath.

- o *By working in this way we can help the Inherent Wisdom of the Blue Print to Surface and the emotions, pain, histories, traumas and stories that were so in the foreground before can get a little smaller. We want to help magnify the Health. *

Settling into Practitioner Neutral and Its Importance in Craniosacral Therapy
- Talk about the Importance for the Practitioner to settle when doing this work.
  - o When listening to the Craniosacral System it is important to stay neutral about what we find in the fascial system.

  - o We want to hold an awareness of the whole system even when we feel pulling in the connective tissue.

  - o We need to be aware of any judgments or assumptions. "One of the reasons it has been so difficult for modern science to study the motions of the Breath of Life is because the system is so intelligent it knows when it is being watched that it will act accordingly."(James Jealous, OD) So, we must maintain a neutral state for the inherent health in the client to surface.

  - o Also, people are most orientated to their traumas, dysfunctions, chronic pain, etc anyways. It is a part of our job as a professional in the healing arts to help the body remember the health that it there, even in the face of chronic pain, trauma, illness, disease and injury. The patterns of organization in the body are always operating to find homeostasis so even when there is unbalance there is health.

- *One of the ways to cultivate practitioner neutral is to maintain stillness while listening to the craniosacral system, keep the awareness wide and not to get pulled into a clients system too much when you notice something. Allow what is there to come to you. Don't go looking for imbalances. Realize the Health with a capital H.*

o **Being-ness in the Presence of a Client:** Settling Exercise with partner (exploring Being-ness in the presence of a client) – have students pair up and face on another in a comfortable sitting position – Begin with eyes closed and settling into their own body – Then have practitioner open their eyes looking at the client while maintaining a sense of their own body. *(Activity) optional*

V. **Clinical Application: Stages in the Inherent Treatment Plan**
1. The practitioner
   a. Enters a state of presence, a being state
   b. Orients to Primary Respiration in his or her own system
   c. Orients to primary respiration relative in the clients system
   d. Orients to and deepens into Dynamic Stillness from which the Breath of Life and primary respiration arise
   e. Establishes and negotiates a safe relational field in a wide field of awareness (wide perceptual field)

f. Has the ability to sense primary respiration oriented to the clients mid-line and system in a wide perceptual field

2. The settling of the relational field.
    - Which entails the process of basic trust emerging as the clients settles into a session. No depth of healing can take place without this safe therapeutic atmosphere similar to what was explained in establishing Practitioners Neutral.

3. The settling and shift of orientation of the clients system from conditional patterns and nervous system activation to wholeness and primary respiration – Holistic Shift.

4. The emergence of healing intensions and processes from levels of Mid-tide, Long Tide or Dynamic Stillness.

5. The resolution of inertia and traumatic forces and patterns.

6. Commonly finishing with a phase of re-orientation of the system to natural mid-lines and re-organization of the fluid and tissue fields to natural fulcrums.

Integration: Before and After a hands-on session:

Verbal Dialogue with Clients = Reflective Mirroring Technique

Note: Because of the subtly of this work it can be important to help facilitate the client in being present with their body sensations before and after a session.

o Seated – Centering, Body Scan (physical body, emotional body, mental body, spiritual body) Intention for the session (Reflect Back= Feedback exactly what you hear back to the client. Do Not add your own words; simply repeat back what you heard.) *Lead client through the centering mediation then ask them what their goal or intension is for the session. Repeat back what you heard.*

- During the session – if needed – What happening Now? Tell Me More? Feed it Back *by Repeating back what you heard*

  o Integration – Have client come back to an upright position.

  o Acknowledgement – practitioner states what they sincerely want to honor to the client.

Ethics note:

Important Note: The trick to safe ethical dialogue during session is to simply repeat back what the client says. This is called the Reflective Mirroring Technique. Do not interject words, thoughts or ideas that are not the clients. Sometimes because the nature of craniosacral therapy people can have the occasional emotional release, if this happens you can ask what is happening now but only repeat what you hear them say do not offer advice. If need be refer the client to a psychologist if they need someone to talk things out with them. We only use dialogue to help them integrate their own experiences of the work into their attention or consciousness. It is not our job to tell them anything.

It is important to avoid the psychological arena when giving osteopathic treatments of Craniosacral Therapy. The movement of the Breath of Life and Primary Respiration alone is what preserves the transformation process of the psychology. Psycho-therapeutic dialogue is not essential to the therapeutic process of the inherent treatment plan and can be more of an interruption to the therapeutic process.

How to conduct a session

A. Begin with Client Seated – Centering Body Scan and Intention (FIB)
B. Begin session at the feet – wait for client neutral
C. Treat what make sense to you (use what happening now and tell me more)
D. Finish at the feet or sacrum
E. Integration – have client come back to a seated position – what stood out? How does this relate to life? Inner wisdom? Affirmation? Action? (FIB) *Optional*
F. Acknowledgement

The essence of what is mysterious and magical in the universe is the same essence of which our bodies grow around in utero.

A. Precautions/Contraindications

This gentle approach is extremely safe in most cases. However, craniosacral therapy is not recommended in cases of acute systemic infections, recent skull fracture, recent spinal tap or puncture to the craniosacral system, intracranial hemorrhage, aneurysm, stroke or herniation of the medulla oblongata (brain stem). Craniosacral therapy does not preclude the use of other medical approaches. Refer to an advanced therapist, or proceed after the client's physician verifies things are ok and gives you the go-ahead.

Chapter Twelve

The Physics of Health

The body is a map of consciousness. We hold every experience within the physical tissues of our bodies. Once the body has experienced a particular event there will forever remain a remnant of that experience somewhere within the muscle and tissue memory. The importance to self healing lies deep within the interrelation of the emotional and physical patterns that manifest within the body as a direct mirror of inner consciousness. Disturbances in health can cause disturbances in intellect. Confliction in the emotional realm will also manifest itself in the tissues of the physical body. This type of connectivity is crucial to understand where the source of true healing comes from.

One of the amazing things about the body is that it knows at all times what it needs to be healthy. What is so ground breaking in this analogy, is that it is scientifically understood through Osteopathic medicine, Chinese medicine and Ayurvedic medicine. These sciences acknowledge that by recognizing the deepest of our soul intention as a direct manifestation of life force energy, which can actually be palpated as the Breath of Life inherent within the cerebrospinal fluid and cell metabolism, we can help the body release physical and emotional holding patterns and get it to remember its own inherent health. By rewiring the nervous system it is possible to heal from just about any form of trauma, but in order to get there we have to honor all sides of consciousness. The physical, emotional and spiritual bodies do not come one without the other.

The mysteries of every nation taught that the laws, elements and powers of the universe were epitomized within the human constitution. Everything that exists outside has its analogy within. It is a fact that our bodies are unique microcosms possessing a reality of its own, but in order to truly understand this concept we must first explore the anatomy of the universe and the simple laws of existence.

Every physical manifestation in the natural world is involved in some form of consciousness. The physical aspect is like the vehicle for life, while the emotional or conscious aspect is like the driver. Life is bonded by the mutual agreement between the cells. The cells carry a vital intelligence through the process called mitosis, which is where the cells split and multiply. Through this process of mitosis the cells demonstrate the steps of evolution through the act of reincarnation. The cells likewise demonstrate the mysteries of the invisible realm identical to all things that are living. During their method of mitosis, the nuclei, which is the brain of the cell, mysteriously disappears. As the cell begins to split into two parts the nuclei reappears in the new cells. This act of intelligence explains the act of transmutation and how energy and matter are in a constant cycle of transformation. Even the smallest and simplest properties within life are indeed alive and thinking within an aspect of a greater whole.

The Atom is the brain of all that exists and is the ordering force of reality. Yet, science has never seen an Atom. This is because the Atom lives in the invisible realm. We only know it truly exists because when matter collides with anti-matter, the invisible opposite of matter, it creates pure energy in the form of an explosion. We also know that nothing in the universe can exist without its invisible counterpart, the Atom. But how did the first Atom come to be, and what exactly is the invisible counterpart? It would seem that the answer lies within both science and religion. The first explosion of the universe, and all things thereafter, was the rising of consciousness and the intent to live. It would seem that intention is what makes everything throughout the universe. The atom (which I will rename intention), is the center piece of all things and it is its permeation throughout space that make all things a reality.

Energy does not stay in the center it permeates throughout the entire space around it. Just like the life giving sun in our solar system, energy radiates out through the lengths of space to give us the nurturing energy to exist. The source of our healing begins in the center of our own universe, in the atom of intention, which permeates out from its origin.

We are made of pure energy, as everything in the universe is made of energy. Everything is simply vibrating particles of movement creating energy and life. Dynamic patterns of energy bundles, that form molecular structures, only move at speeds making us believe that the world is made of material substance. Energy and matter are interchangeable, for one cannot exist without the other. Just as the mind, body and spirit operate together, intention, energy and matter function as one unit in the laws of existence.

The universe is an interconnected cosmic web, where all things are in a constant flow of change and transformation. The constitutions of matter are all interrelated as integrated parts of a whole. All matter is a transformation of the same matter, for it all comes from the same place. Everything in the universe is made of the same atoms and substances. Energy just simply transforms from one form to another. It does not dissipate, not even in the cell process of mitosis where the nuclei disappears it simple enters into a different realm. We call this phenomenon within the universe *transmutation*, and it can be explained as the journey between life and death, and death and life.

Scientific laws clearly state that all things are a part of an integrated whole. No event is understood as isolated. Intention, in the present form of the atom, is the birthing place of energy and life. All things are in relation to one another through the commonality if intention. We are all connected, and going to the core of understanding helps the outside manifest from the inside.

When we begin to see the world as molecules spinning with the intention to live, we can understand the depth of our experience to a slightly greater degree. The unique intention of the soul's purpose sits underneath the chaotic movement that makes life. Just as the atom lies within the cerebrospinal fluid and the original blue print which gives every cell in the body a means to exist.

Another aspect of universe intelligence includes, that all living matter has a retreating and expanding pattern of movement much like the breath. The Breath of Life, which in inherent in the living energy system of the cerebrospinal fluid, allows the essence of our souls' intention to manifest as an expression of life. Life is a creative, non linear, unfolding event that swells out into the space around it. All aspects of our functioning, individually and as a global community, are an exploration of movement that is an existential and spiritual unfolding.

The cells and tissues of the body naturally align to the universal system through movement, just as the mind does when it is still. The soul of intention lies deep within the stillness of movement, just as the mind does when it is still. The soul of intention lies deep within the stillness of movement, just as the Atom rests quietly within the invisible realm of all matter. All forms of life are organized by stillness, and stillness is necessary for movement to reset and carry out the intention for life.

We call the stillness of life *dynamic stillness*, and it has the ability to bring us back to who we are. It is the quietness that lies just within and center of all movement (within ourselves and all living things) that our original intention can be felt. Stillness is where the soul resides. When we sit in stillness it helps us to remember the intention behind life. Therefore, we can radiate that intention into the cells, without confusion, to help us on the life path of universal consciousness. We all have a role to play in this grand theater called life, and stillness can help us to understand that role. However, to confront the soul, the unique intention of the soul's purpose which sits in the presence of dynamic stillness, can be a very frightening experience; especially, if you are alone and have never done so before. We touch upon it and if like we may be dying, (much like a traumatic experience). Underneath the movement of our cells, our bodies, our minds and our breath there is an intention so still that is also life but it is not driven or understood by anything that is familiar in the third dimensional reality of which our society lives. The intention, behind our reality has a means to exist without bodily functions, can only be described as a feeling, and is the aspect of ourselves that will go on after death. It is quiet and humble, (as it sits), observing the dynamics of life, and it is like a huge and silent statue standing underneath our skin. It is what science would call the Atom of our unique intention and its reality is the aspect of ourselves that will transmute throughout the universe when we are dead.

Movement awareness is the easiest way to still the mind. It provides an outlet to explore the stillness of the soul. Moving keeps us in check, helping us to remember we are alive, creating a safe heaven and diminishing the fear that may be associated with confronting the big silent statue. Then as we become more comfortable looking at the soul, we can drop into stillness more readily in order to feel the soul intention and to figure out how to carry out its wishes.

Spiritual study of the self is the meeting place between the universal and the individual intention. It is this type of journey that will help us towards understanding the core center of our health, and the deep meaning behind our existence. To study the self is to take the courageous road toward holistic health and understanding of the soul. The search for the invisible counterpart is not for the faint of heart, because you have to be willing to look at yourself. If we are not used to feeling the connection we have with the universe, the soul can be a very scary space, especially when you pile traumatic experiences within the body. Touching the soul for the first time can resurrect traumatic memory from past experiences, so in order to safely explore the Atom of intention we must be willing to process old patterns.

All forms of trauma have physiological effects within the body. Old trauma is accompanied with the fight or flight response and retention of the breath. This effect creates a still point within the cerebral spinal fluid and energetically imprints a record of shock within the nervous system. In turn, this creates a marvelous survival mechanism within the muscle memory. Therefore, our bodies will continue to hold traumatic patterns until we can figure out how to release them.

When we carry traumatic experiences it can be detrimental to the way we function in the world. Most of us can understand this when we have been in an accident of some kind where the muscles and bones are permanently damaged. Some of us can understand this through emotional trauma that forever scars the way we relate and interact in the world. Either way when we experience trauma in one respect or another it will also manifest in the opposite system. Emotional trauma to the heart, for instance, will cause us to physically contract the muscles in the chest, and physical trauma from an accident will create emotional imbalances from the shock and fear that took place during a moment when we were vulnerable. Therefore, in order to work trauma out of the body, we have to include both the realms of the physical and emotional. You can not completely release physical trauma without addressing the emotional, and you can not completely release emotional trauma without acknowledging the physical. The two are completely related and cannot be viewed as separate entities.

Incidentally, when using stillness to explore the depths of the soul, the experience of past trauma will arise. What is happening is that the spirit and body are working together to encourage a person to resolve the trauma and integrate new neuro-pathways. This process is preparing the body to let go of fear. It is impossible to glimpse the soul completely with any type of fear within the body. We have to let go of fear and hold nothing but acceptance and loving kindness for the place we are in our lives, in order to peer into the eye of the soul; which can only be done in the realm of unconditional love so that we do not create a traumatic experience because we have refused to look at ourselves. This is a demonstration of vital intelligence and how the body is always operating in a wholistic realm. (We must remember that the mind, body and spirit operate as one unit, just as the Atom, energy and matter function together in the laws of Physics; the Atom relating to the spirit, energy to the mind, and matter to the body.) In order to work directly with the soul it is important to realize that one must confront the dramas that have conditioned us along the path of life. These dramas are not out true selves. They are masks of identity that fool us into thinking that we are the way we are, just as the movement of the cells fool us into thinking the world is solid. By looking at the soul, the Atom of intention, we can free ourselves from karmic experiences that were induced by traumas. And we do that by first working out old patterns we have in the body. Through the connectivity between mind/body/spirit, we penetrate the depth of our soul through exploration of the physical and emotional expressions that we carry. This is how the body is a map of consciousness, and why it is important to recognize the connection in order to understand where true healing comes from.

True healing and the ability to live life of self realization entails hard work. It incorporates a path where you are in constant occupation with all the aspects of self. You cannot live in denial on the road to healing. You have to be prepared to be confronted by your worst fears, and to understand that as soon as healing occurs you may be confronted with a challenge, that your soul self will initiate in order to help facilitate a new pattern of growth. That is why being familiar with the soul is helpful in order to stay grounded and stable, along the life path. The potential for trauma is always present, but if we remain present with our souls' intention we can operate our free will towards the path that lays closest to the heart. This is why healing the whole person, not just the ailing part, is the only way to achieve true healing.

We have to peel away the sheaths of our existence in order to get to the soul. The physical, mental, intellectual, and energetic sheaths are like layers that surround the spirit sheath. That is why when we touch the soul for the first time, it can create a traumatic experience. In order to understand our unique Atom of intention, we have to work through the outer sheaths. Then as the work becomes clearer, we can express our impact on humanity in a way that is non-conditional by society, judgment or traumatic experiences. Rather, we can work in a way that is in direct communication with the universal source and the heart of our own unique intention.

Walking the path to complete health is a very scary road. It is very hard to do alone, because it requires us to look at our soul and to question the real reason behind illness and pain. In order to heal we have to muster up the courage to confront the soul, but we must do it in the most loving way imaginable. Because when we are void of love it is impossible to heal. Hatred, skepticism and self doubt have no place in the healing process and make it impossible to heal. You have to believe you can heal and sometimes you need people to support you.

As science proves the facts of the human condition, touch therapy is becoming more and more important. Support in the form of loving touch is irreplaceable when it comes to trauma and illness. Babies and young children die without loving touch, which should be a reminder to reach out compassionately towards all people that are living in this world.

We are made of energy and bound to each other through the interconnected web of the field that surrounds us. Even a thought of hatred could deeply hurt a person. Feelings, DNA, matter and emotions also have a vibrational sound quality to them. In fact, all life forms produce their own sound frequency. Even our planet Earth has a heart beat that is the sound of the vibrational OM. Our own unique sound is the echo of the heartbeat, breath, cerebral spinal fluid, cell mitosis and all the functions of the organs. All movement within the body makes a sound. Even our brainwaves and DNA sing. This fact, (that we hold song), should be a reminder for when we interact with other people; because the feelings we hold towards ourselves and others will radiate into other peoples frequency. This is due to the fact that we are connected through the cosmic web, which binds us together energetically.

All things possess vital intelligence manifest in various forms of movement, through an expansion and contraction breath, which follows along the vibrational intention present within the DNA and the core existence of your own unique intention. We cannot live life alone and in isolation forever, because the need for human support is essential to our heath and healing process. True healing and self realization comes from the exploration of the self, which entails working through old traumas. Dynamic stillness is where the soul sits in contemplation, and it is where we must go in order to reset the neuro-pathways of the physical self. The body is a map of consciousness which possesses all the physical laws of the universe.

And, we must honor all the things that happen to us in our lives because experiences are our greatest source of learning.

About the Author

Dominique Clothiaux's journey into Biodynamic Craniosacral Therapy began at a very young age. From the age of 5 years old she suffered from debilitating migraines. It was her mother, a pediatric physical therapist who gave her first Craniosacral therapy treatments for many years until the migraines resolved at the age of 11. As an adult she became a manual therapist. Fascinated with Craniosacral therapy, she set out to study with every imaginable Craniosacral therapist available in the united states. The main focus of her work for over two decades has been focused on how to subtly release deep tensions centered around the central nervous system by facilitating Stillness.

Registered Craniosacral Therapist® with the Biodynamic Craniosacral Therapy Association of North America, Approved Continuing Education Provider with the National Certification Board of Massage and Bodywork, Pre and Perinatal Birth Educator through The Kutenai Institute of Integral Therapies, Virginia State Licensed Massage Therapist, Neonatal Resuscitation Provider. She has taught a foundational course in Biodynamic Craniosacral Therapy nationally since 2007. As a Craniosacral and Manual Therapist Dominique has conducted over 10,000 sessions.

Today Dominique practices as *a Licensed Midwife by the Virginia Board of Medicine & a Certified Professional Midwife (CPM) with the North American Registry of Midwives (NARM)*. As a Midwife, she has attended nearly 650 births and specialize in out-of-hospital birth. Her vision is to protect the sanctity of physiological birth and to help foster the understanding and importance about the Primal Health Period.

Dominique can be reached at www.birthandbiodynamics.com

www.ingramcontent.com/pod-product-compliance
Lightning Source LLC
Chambersburg PA
CBHW072158290526
45794CB00004B/1562